THE NUTCRACKER IS ALREADY DANCING

THE NUTCRACKER IS ALREADY DANCING

The HIVs and the HIV-Nots

CARY SAVITCH M.D.

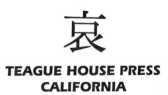

TEAGUE HOUSE PRESS
CALIFORNIA

The Nutcracker Is Already Dancing
The HIVs and the HIV-Nots

By Cary Savitch, M.D.

Published By: **Teague House Press**, P.O. Box 24258, Ventura, California 93002 U.S.A.

Publisher's Cataloging-in-Publication
  (Prepared by Quality Books Inc.)
Savitch, Cary.
  The Nutcracker is already dancing : the HIVs and HIV-nots / Cary Savitch
  p. cm.
  Includes bibliographical references and index.
  Preassigned LCCN: 96-90495
  ISBN 0-9653697-5-7

  1. AIDS (Disease) 2. AIDS (Disease)—Social aspects. 3. HIV infections. I. Title

RA644.A25S38 1996   362.1'969792
                           QBI96-40207

Printed in the United States of America
10 9 8 7 6 5 4 3 2

Book design by Karla Haeberle
Cover design and illustration by Armgardt Design

WARNING-DISCLAIMER

The views expressed in this book are solely those of the author. They do not necessarily represent the opinions of anyone else who has contributed to this book.

Statistics were obtained from multiple sources including personal communications. Since HIV screening is incomplete, many referenced sources substituted extrapolations for actual numbers. The author has tried to be as accurate as possible in lending interpretation to the data available. Information is provided only up until the date of printing.

This book is released with the understanding that the publisher and author are not engaged here in rendering individual medical advice. Many aspects of AIDS will continue to remain controversial. As such, individual questions pertaining to treatment and diagnosis are referred to the reader's own health care provider.

The author shares many personal experiences. Names and locations have been altered except when those individuals involved insisted it was not necessary. Because the AIDS epidemic is so widespread some readers might recognize similarities to people and experiences in their own lives. These similarities are coincidental, perhaps acting to bring us closer together in understanding the human tragedy of AIDS.

This book is dedicated to my uncle, Marty Yudson, who died of colon cancer in 1992. He believed in a higher level of humor in the face of adversity.

EIGHT BLUNDERS

Out of these grows the violence that plagues the world:

Wealth without work

Pleasure without conscience

Knowledge without character

Commerce without morality

Science without humanity

Worship without sacrifice

Politics without principles

Rights without responsibilities

— *Mahatma Gandhi, 1947*

CONTENTS

PREFACE

No person or pill will save you. Every God has been approached. Every prayer has gone unanswered.

The moment it takes you to read this sentence someone new will be infected with HIVirus. Someone just like yourself will develop AIDS and die. Today's children have a greater chance of dying of AIDS than of heart disease or cancer. Estimates indicate that 10,000 new cases of HIV infection are acquired daily throughout the world. This disease cannot be cured.

During my early years of medical training, if anyone had ever told me that there would someday exist a new contagious disease that would be universally lethal and kill millions of people, and that efforts would be made *not* to identify those infected, I would have thought that situation insane. Today I am witness to this insanity. Sadly, I am also a participant.

Blood was once symbolic of life. Today it is tainted. Likewise, our lives have been tainted with distrust. Greater importance is placed on sexual preference than on human preservation. The most dangerous epidemic of modern time, and possibly of all time, is being fought with swords of individual rights and shields of privacy. Only the human spirit is being defeated.

I have treated patients with AIDS since 1981. My efforts and those of others have consistently met with failure. Each year the trauma intensifies as the avalanche of death gains momentum. Might this cease only when there is no one left to infect?

I did not have the luxury of a retreat or sabbatical while writing this book. The words and paragraphs were interrupted by patient care. This further served to remind me of the importance of telling the story as I see it and live it.

I could never have written this book without the experience and privilege of treating patients with AIDS. It was not by plan that my involvement started during the first days of this epidemic. During the course of writing this book I have shared personal experiences from 1978 through 1996 that have shaped my thinking about this disease. My perceptions have shifted with the evolution of this epidemic. I now challenge medical consensus to which I once ascribed.

Many of the people in this book, along with their friends and family, I came to know well. They shared the darkest and most tragic moments of their lives with me. Their stories and their case histories will continue to live with me. Names have been changed, although many families insisted this was not necessary. The events are real. They come from medical records, and what was left in my memory and stored in my heart.

During the writing of this book I exercise an occasional play on words. There is no intention of offending any person or group. This choice is a necessary ingredient to humanize this tragedy and arouse public attention. It also serves to maintain my sanity. Millions of people dying in the AIDS holocaust are going unnoticed and forgotten.

Many AIDS infected people live in despair. Someone infected them. Someone passed them the poison without the antidote. "If no one cares about me, why should I care?" Many of them separate their own fate from the fate of the human race. Without conscience, death is spread to a lover or a stranger. Identification with the human family is lost. The time for mending is in order.

Why did I write this book? In simple terms, it is something I had to do. AIDS has been my train wreck. I have saved no one, yet I am considered an expert. My colleagues have done no better. My family is on the train. It is time to speak out!

I wish this text could be more uplifting. Instead it tells the truth as I see it. It is a story of despair: the personal failure of my efforts to cure anyone, public health's failure to contain this epidemic, and society's failure to become involved. What I have written is exactly what I believe.

AIDS education is flawed and failing. The principles of epidemiology that apply to all communicable diseases have been broken, ignored, and even ridiculed. We have yet to practice appropriate prevention. We have yet to practice the infection control measures I have been taught as a medical student. By remaining silent I share the blame.

Is the AIDS epidemic containable? Yes! It is within our capability to identify everyone infected and restrict further transmission. However, a time is reached beyond which even prevention is too late. Will we continue on the same path of waiting for the miracle cure while watching millions more die? Do we have the courage as a society to do what is imperative now to curb the spread of this virus? How many lives are we willing to sacrifice at the altar of civil rights? The reader will participate in making these decisions, by action or by default.

There is no solace in criticizing any individual, organization, or institution. I share my uncompromised version of a public health tragedy. The goal is a call to action. We must breathe life into public health services. The unleashed power referred to by ACT-UP (AIDS Coalition To Unleash Power) must focus on prevention. Activist groups, with purposeful social agenda, are challenging medical reality and scientific truths. This book is my response to that challenge.

It is natural for me to feel sensitive regarding how others will accept my ideas. The extreme right may perceive me as a gay sympathizer. They will be correct. I am empathetic to the plight of the gay community and the threat of its extinction. Some among the radical gay left may view me as an outsider, one who does not represent gay ideology. They will also be correct. My purpose is beyond conforming to anyone else's ideology. I am only trying, objectively, to relate how a small virus is impacting man's ability to survive.

I expect knee-jerk criticism for promoting a position that argues for universal HIV testing and mandatory reporting of all test results to public health officials. In addition to education and counseling, stringent public health policies must include intervention whenever and wherever necessary to curb the AIDS epidemic. Many people are not prepared for a radical change of thinking and action. We rely on rules and regulations instead of common sense to control this epidemic. Every current effort to control AIDS is failing.

Public chastisement is anticipated from some in the medical community who still cling to the erroneous dogma that has surrounded this epidemic. I once shared the myth. Those academicians and educators who do not directly treat patients may underestimate the personal pain and frustration surrounding each AIDS diagnosis. Most do not write the prescriptions for drugs that only pretend to work. Some may not fully comprehend the global consequences of never having a vaccine or the human suffering of never having a cure. They do not sign the death certificates!

The medical community has miscalculated the extent of the failure of public health services. I challenge the political conscience that has defined public health policy. We have abandoned our concern for the safety and protection of the uninfected. In an epidemic of this proportion it is not heretical to show concern for the uninfected. The minimal response of health care agencies to a deadly pathogen completely out of control is not acceptable. The meager effort to prevent transmission warrants explanation. Currently the control of AIDS rests in the hands (and hearts) of those who are HIV-infected. It is my conviction that a social change is inevitable if mankind is to endure this pandemic.

All too often clinicians do not balance the responsibility they have to their patients with the inherent responsibility owed to the well being of society. A good doctor addresses the medical needs of the patient. But a good doctor does not protect the privacy of the patient at the risk of endangering the lives of others.

There is sharp disagreement among health care providers, activists, civil libertarians, and all concerned citizens about how to respond to the AIDS crisis. There is no consensus as to whether we are making progress, faltering on the edge of an abyss, or have already plunged beyond rescue. I hope to provide some common ground of understanding based on my own personal and clinical experiences.

Statistics contained in this text originate primarily from government sources. Most figures are extrapolations from data that is incomplete since testing is not currently required and reporting is haphazard. Numbers pass from medical conference to medical conference, journal to journal, with little verification. The criteria presently used to identify a new case of AIDS does little more than uncover who was infected five to fifteen years ago.

When the sun rises tomorrow morning there will still be no cure for AIDS. Cure means to eradicate the virus from the body and eliminate any chance of transmission. There may never be a vaccine. Prevention of transmission is man's only hope to control the AIDS epidemic. That hope is time limited and it is being squandered.

Many concerned patients, colleagues, and friends, who have encouraged me to complete this text, have asked who the audience I hoped to reach will be. Students? Physicians? Worried parents? Political leaders? Educators? I have narrowed the readership to only two groups, those who are infected and those who are not.

My story is personal. I fear for my own three children who will face an untamed virus. This fear must be harnessed into a plan of action that aims at prevention. The alternative will be unprecedented social chaos. The success or failure of this book can only be measured by how it affects the intensity of this epidemic.

Readers who choose to use this text as a reference must recognize that it is written from one viewpoint. My beliefs are not necessarily shared by my colleagues or by the institutions where I trained, at least not yet. Readers are urged to seek information beyond what is contained here and debate every controversial assertion. Keep the dialogue alive. Formulate your own opinions. Participate in your own destiny.

Our ability to survive a major change in the environment, including a new predator virus, will ultimately be determined by how much we love each other, not by how much we fear each other.

The uninfected cannot forever remain unaffected.

— Cary Savitch, M.D.

JUST SCRATCHING THE SURFACE

1

Little drops of rain, whisper of the pain,
tears of love's lost in the days gone by. . .
Upon us all a little rain must fall.

— Led Zeppelin

L ove and fear can come from the same heart. It scared your family. James, it scared me.

I stopped every drug you were on but it didn't help the itching. Topical creams all failed. You couldn't stop scratching your arms. This caused a constant oozing from bloody scabs.

When I watch baseball I think of you. I remember your telling me of your nephew who won baseball's coveted Cy Young pitching award. You were just as proud of your grandson who played jr. varsity football at the local high school. Every time I wear the Hawaiian shirt your daughter sewed for me I also think of you, your bleeding arms, and your wonderful family.

In 1980 you retired from the military at age 53. The following year you were transfused one unit of blood at Wadsworth V.A. Hospital in Los Angeles when your heart valve was replaced. If the surgery had been performed in North Dakota or some other area where HIVirus was not as prevalent you might be alive today. **Blood in Los Angeles in 1981 was not safe.** You were transfused in a vulnerable year in a vulnerable city. It was recommended that you be screened for HIV when the test was eventually made available. This was part of the "look-back study" set up cooperatively by blood banks. This was one of the few correct efforts made on behalf of public safety. Fortunately this program escaped the accusing scream of "discrimination" from activist groups. Your retirement did not go as planned—no boat, no cabin, no camp outs with the grandchildren.

The pruritis (itching) began in 1986. Other symptoms followed. Your wife was with you at each office visit. This woman was a saint. You were enrolled in a study that treated you monthly with passive immuno-globulin donated by other infected patients. Together we tried every conventional and unconventional means of therapy.

The fear we all had of your weeping arms was real. This was nothing you could do anything about. It created an anxiety for your children and heightened their concern about you being around the young grandchildren. I know you understood, but still felt the pain. They loved you as much as you loved them.

Your wife still visits with me. She is just as charming as ever. She tests HIV-negative and cherishes every moment with your grandchildren.

ICE AIDS: IN THE END

*There are times when one would like to
hang the whole human race,
and finish the farce.*

— Mark Twain

The dinosaur roamed this planet as *king* for 140 million years. One explanation for their extinction is a shower of large meteorites or asteroids that struck the earth 66 million years ago. This resulted in fire storms destroying vegetation and creating dust clouds that blocked the sun's rays. This blanket of debris kept the surface of the earth cool, further depleting the dinosaurs' food supply. The dinosaur was put to rest after many millions of years of dominant survival. Even these great creatures could not adjust forever to the dynamically changing environment.

Homosapiens have lived in delicate balance with other living species, both plant and animal, for 1.1 million years. If man's existence could be extended an additional 300,000 years beyond the present, humans could claim to have survived a period of time equal to 1% of the time the dinosaur survived. It is unlikely that humankind is suited to ever be that successful. The environment is in continual flux. Four different species become extinct on earth each hour, partially as a result of one species, man. Over 99% of all species that have ever existed on earth are already extinct. New species are continually given the opportunity to claim a place in the ecosystem. Some species lay dormant, only to eventually resurface under more favorable circumstances.

There have been five mass extinctions on Earth over the past 800 million years. Some archeologists believe the Earth may presently be in the midst of a sixth major mass extinction. It began when Ice Age hunters began to wipe out the megafauna. It continues today through habitat destruction and human interference.

Currently a certain new predator is in town. It may have been forced out from the rain forest by man's intrusion. This viral species may have been in existence among humans in millenniums past, adapting poorly but continually trying to re-emerge. Modern man has made its task easy. DNA imprinting even suggests that nonfunctioning retroviral nucleic acid may already exist in the human genetic code. A possible distant cousin of prior retroviruses has resurfaced.

The HIVirus is not challenging to be a new king, but it is certainly capable of dethroning man. This small speck of RNA also requires man for its own survival. This particular virus does not successfully replicate outside the human host. The symbiosis with man is nature's play. If every human being were to be infected, the virus would likely perish as well. The human species can live without this little fellow but it cannot live without man—advantage, humans.

At question is how important is human survival to humans? How willing are we to adapt to a new environment that we created, and that includes a smart new species? This adaptation will necessarily require a change in human behavior, in a real sense, a human mutation.

DOMINAIDS

The trigger is drawn, and the hammer is down
And the hour glass is running out.
There is no turning back the hands of the clock.
— Jimmy Cliff

L ike dominoes they fell. First it was Leonard . . . then it was Christine. . . then it was Leonard's wife, Anita. . . then it was Anita's new husband.

Leonard was looking for a new start in life. His drug problem, as long as he stayed in New York City, would not go away. He had resorted to prostituting men to support his habit. He was married to Anita, who had a brother living in California. To save their marriage and to save Leonard's life, they would move west—as far from Hell's Kitchen and the heroin shooting galleries as possible. There was only one thing they couldn't leave behind them. *It was silently replicating in Leonard's body.* This was 1980. I was still in San Francisco completing an Infectious Disease Fellowship. Our paths would first cross three years later.

It is now 1983. Leonard has a good job in sales management. He has survived heroin and Hepatitis B. He can certainly survive as the manager of a major department store chain. He knows how to schmooze.

He has given up smoking. Why the cough now?

First it was the white tongue and swollen lymph nodes in his neck. His weight was difficult to maintain. His cough and shortness of breath worried Anita the most. His chest x-ray showed diffuse bilateral interstitial pneumonia. In the evening the hospital pathologist and I reviewed the special silver methenamine stains made on the bronchial washings obtained earlier in the day. Pneumocystis. I would inform Leonard and Anita the following morning. There was no HIV test available in 1983. The retrovirus to be implicated as the cause of AIDS (Acquired Immune Deficiency Syndrome) had not yet been discovered. A brief and partial recovery from his pneumonia was short lived. Leonard died six weeks later.

Christine's headaches would not go away. Days of pain extended to weeks. She went to her doctor. The lumbar puncture confirmed meningitis. An India Ink prep of the spinal fluid showed large encapsulated yeast. Cryptococcus. I was asked to consult.

Christine was 24 years old, just married. By her bedside sat her husband. He would faithfully stay by her side for the next two years. Her soft expression reminded me of my cousin Cheryl. A painful relationship was about to develop.

The Elisa screen of her blood for HIV was positive. I was stunned. When the Western Blot antibody test also came back positive I requested it be repeated at an outside laboratory. The results were the same. Christine and I needed to talk.

"I was just a summer temp," I could remember her lament. She was not promiscuous. Before marriage Christine had one long-term boyfriend. They had occasional sex. Neither had prior sex. She continued to tell me her story but there would be only *one name* that would tell it all. Five years ago, between her freshman and sophomore years in college, she had worked as a temporary sales clerk in a department store. It was there she met someone. He was an assistant manager and quite a bit older than she. "But it was only once." I asked her to tell me his first name. *"Leonard,"* was her response. We never discussed this again. I never told her I knew this man. I didn't need to add to her pain.

Christine moved to Bakersfield, California, when her husband's job was transferred there. Once a week they drove three hours each way to keep her appointments with me. She vowed to fight. She waged a heroic two year battle.

Christine founded the first AIDS support group in Bakersfield.

Anita now works for a cardiologist. Two years after her husband Leonard died, the HIV test became available. I recommended she be tested. She informed me she felt well. I did not see her again until 1988 when I was asked to evaluate a woman who was hospitalized with pneumonia, the same Anita, but with a different last name. Sitting up in her hospital bed she politely said hello as we exchanged greetings. She was now remarried. David, her new husband, appeared several years younger than she and in good health. Anita's life was back in order, so she thought. Anita did a little better than Leonard. She was depleted of all helper T-cells, but lasted about four months.

The next time I saw David was 1994. He looked a shell of his former self. He too suffered the ravages of AIDS — about
       to
           fall!

FROM SALZBURG TO MELSBACH

4

An uncommon act of human decency may have saved my life. He was a stranger who would pass with the night. He was a young German man, an auto accident victim who had sustained a bloody head injury. He also had AIDS, yet he was a person with the courage to alert people who stopped to help him that he was HIV-positive.

But first, let me digress. . . Schillerlocken comes from the belly of a shark-like fish found in the cold waters of the Mosel and Rhine Rivers of Europe. People cut the belly into thin strips and smoke it before eating. The name is given to this fish because, after smoking, it looks like the curled hairs of Friedrich Schiller, a famous 18th century dramatist and poet. German legend also tells of Schiller consuming large quantities of this fish. I was introduced to this delicacy in the summer of 1972 while camping with my friend, Hans, along the banks of the Mosel.

It was a hot morning in July of 1972. I was traveling by myself, the lone American on a packed ferry boat delivering scores of young German vacationers to the sun-scorched beaches of Majorca, one of the Spanish owned Balearic

Islands located in the Mediterranean Sea. I kept hearing the Germans say "Spitz. . . .Spitz" over and over again, referring to the American swimmer, Mark Spitz. He was in Munich that same week totaling record numbers of gold medals in the Olympic games. I remember the scattered beer bottles and the mounds of backpacks on the ship's deck. I can still hear the laughter and singing. The songs were English, the accents were German.

A tall, lanky German of about my age (I later learned we were born five days apart) stared over at me from a guard rail on the ferry. His face was sunburned beyond safe levels and his lean body was slightly stooped. The smile was genuine. Hans befriended me and invited me to join his group of friends. We spent the next week together at a beach resort village on Majorca, occupied almost entirely by Germans. The little Spanish I spoke was rarely needed, as it seemed everyone in that part of Spain was speaking German.

In 1972 Hans was an economics major at the University of Essen in Germany. Today he is a journalist. I was between my third and fourth years of medical school at the University of California, San Francisco. I had just completed a cardiology externship at Hammersmith Hospital in London. Stumbling upon the luxury of six open weeks to travel, I chose to get lost in Europe. I had good health, little money, and a functioning thumb.

Before my return to the States and before Hans needed to be back in classes, we agreed to meet up in Germany. We traveled in his pale blue Citroen Duck, the less expensive French substitute for the German Volkswagen Beetle. Most of our time was spent along the banks of the Mosel River, from where we were able to observe in the distance the famous Seven Mountain Peaks, "The Siebengebirge," that overlooked the Rhine Valley. We spent our time in small villages and campsites along the river edge, visited old castles, and consumed every variety of local wine. Vineyards lined the course of the entire river. Mostly we just talked and built a lasting friendship. We pledged to meet again someday at the same river edge with our families, and to always keep in touch.

The following year, 1973, Hans and his friend, Rainer, came to visit California. We backpacked together at Yosemite National Park. In 1975 I briefly saw Hans in Germany before extending my travels to Ghana.

It was a morning in late May of 1994. My children were bumping and howling through the ritual rush to school. Calling their good-byes as they rushed out the kitchen door I rescued and finished their three soggy bowls of cereal. Was it fatigue from being on call the night before or was it the 22 years since I had last tasted Schillerlocken? I did miss seeing Hans. We kept in touch by postcards, letters, and pictures. For 14 years my wife had been asking me who was this "Hans guy!" She kept sending him annual Christmas pictures of our family. Hans observed my three children grow up, but they had never met. Only I knew Hans. It was time to visit. It was time to make good on a pledge made by both of us. When I telephoned him it had been 19 years since I had last heard his voice.

Hans now lives with his family in Melsbach, Germany. This is a small village several miles from the town of Neuwied, which means "new river" in German. The community sits along the Rhine River twenty-eight miles downstream from Koblenz, where the Mosel meets the Rhine. As smoothly as those two rivers join, our families came together as Hans and I did 22 years earlier. We visited the very same sites along the Mosel where Hans and I had once camped. The Schillerlocken was less plentiful and a lot more oily than I had remembered. I needed only a taste to put me back in time.

I was touched that every photograph, card, and letter ever sent to Hans was kept in his living room in a special folder designated for my family. He and his family already knew my children through pictures and vacation postcards. We got along wonderfully and they have since visited us in California.

After spending time with Hans in Germany, my family and I crammed into a medium-sized, non-air-conditioned rental car to continue our journey. My daughter, Jessica, kept reminding me how cheap I was to rent a car without air-conditioning in 100 degree weather. Everyone agreed with her, including myself by the end of the trip. My two boys did not want to leave Hans and his magic tricks. From Germany we traveled south to Tuscany, then through the Italian Alps into Austria.

Prior to leaving Hans, we promised to see him before our return flight home. This now meant traveling from Salzburg to Melsbach, 681 km, in seven hours. We didn't have time on our side, but we did have the German Autobahn, one of the fastest commuter highways in the world. It was also one of the most dangerous, more dangerous than I would have ever thought. Four weeks had passed since I had given any thought to my Infectious Disease practice, being covered back home by my associate.

My holiday would end late that last night before returning home. Tired and cramped into the back seat of a shrinking Nissan, with their souvenirs crushed between them, my children fought each other to sleep. My wife in the passenger seat was already asleep. I was racing 130 km per hour and barely keeping up with the flow of traffic, which fortunately was thinning out through the hot, humid night. Villages, towns, and cities, all with strange names, passed through the darkness. The only breeze was created by our car.

Several blinking red lights and smoking flares interrupted the dark silence. Cars were scattered across the autobahn, pointing in different directions. All traffic was stopped. The ambulances and paramedics had not yet arrived. I got out of our car to help. I was the second motorist at the accident scene. The first was a German truck driver who spoke some English. He was wearing work gloves that were covered with blood. He informed me that one of the accident victims, hunched over in the dark alongside the road and holding his head, had just informed him of being HIV-positive. I was warned to be very careful. I was grateful to have been warned!

In T-shirt and shorts, I was standing sockless, protected only by the soles of my travel-worn sneakers. This was the only barrier to the pooled infected blood and shards of glass crunching under my feet. All the injured appeared to be stable. I carefully walked over to the young man slumped along the roadside, who, fortunately for me, was alert and able to speak. He was holding a towel to his bleeding scalp. He once again warned of his HIV status. He assured me he was okay. I stayed with him until the ambulance arrived. He was lucky he was not injured worse.

I often reflect upon the circumstances of my friendship with Hans, of that holiday, of that night, and of that accident. It was good fortune the young man did not lose consciousness. It was I who was lucky that he was not injured worse.

ONE STRIKE AND YOU'RE OUT

I shall have much more to say when I am dead.
— *Edwin Arlington Robinson*
(John Brown)

5

One wrong swing with the wrong partner and it's over. If you are HIV-negative, *freeze!* Think. Stay alive. **AIDS is no cause worth dying for.**

Each patient helplessly tries to reverse his or her tragedy. AIDS membership is easy. AIDS membership is for life. Once infected, always infected. To quit is to die!

AIDS is associated with a painful and prolonged death. The physical trauma is compounded by a social stigma that often leads to rejection by family and friends. Many patients I treat suffer this fate. Jason's mother publicly proclaimed her son had a brain tumor. I first met her at his burial. Thanksgiving dinner at Roger's went nearly unattended. It would be his last family supper. Marta's parents wished to be notified, but "only after she died." Larry lived in a car for three months, his only companions, a Golden Retriever and tuberculosis.

Patients have pleaded with me not to include AIDS on their death certificate for fear it would show up in their obituary. I know of no other disease where patients continue to suffer even after death. These untouchable victims of HIV often contemplate and commit suicide. The suicide rate is 25 times higher than for the general population. In despair some physicians have assisted in this suicide effort to relieve pain and suffering and unbearable emotional torment.

The only lives that can be saved in this epidemic will be those who are not yet infected. Public health policy must be directed with this clear recognition. Policies must be in place (but presently are not) to include mandatory screening and reporting, and vigorous case contact finding. The primary goal of public health agencies is to contain infectious epidemics. Broad recommendations without teeth don't work against communicable diseases. The practice of epidemiology (the science that studies the incidence, distribution and control of disease in a population) that has been successfully applied to other contagious diseases must be resurrected. The alternative to prevention could be a fragmented human species dying off somewhere into the 21st century. Are we reserving a place on our own endangered species list?

AIDS is a national disaster for America. Every medical response is disappointing. The complete lack of concern for public safety is a disgrace. More Americans will die of AIDS this year alone than have died from all natural disasters, including earthquakes, floods, tornadoes, and hurricanes combined over the past 20 years. AIDS is the leading cause of death in the gay population. Nothing else comes close. More young gay men die of AIDS than from the next seven leading causes of death added together (excluding accidents). Twenty-five years old is now considered middle age in the gay male population. The combination of an intelligent, deadly virus and a host sapped of common sense spells grave consequences for decades to come.

AIDS has a global complexion. Health policies regarding this disease must be universally acceptable. No people or countries are immune to this pathogen. Protection and survival for any one nation requires international control or self-imposed isolation. Any deadly emerging virus can be transported to any part of the world within 20 hours. The

AIDS virus has already crossed every border.

The United States is looked upon for leadership. This nation's influence must take into account the unique political, demographic, and economic differences of other regions. General agreements acceptable to every nation must be reached. All scientific information must be shared and scrutinized. The epidemic knows no boundaries. Any new case anywhere on the planet affects the entire human family.

The challenge for cooperation has never been greater. The threat of this tiny retrovirus, just like the threat of nuclear war, is proof that "We Are One."

THE OAKLAND AIDS BRIDGE MEETS THE GOLDEN GAY BRIDGE

And in the naked light I saw...10,000 people maybe more.
People talking without speaking. People hearing without listening.
People writing songs that voices never shared.
No one dared. . .disturb the sound of silence.

6

— *Paul Simon (The Sounds of Silence)*

The original "Buds Ice Cream," located in lower Castro, is what I remember best.

I had no clue. I often wonder if there was prophecy in the musical lyrics of Paul Simon. Could he or anyone have known that the world would soon witness 10,000 new HIV infections everyday? The silence would soon be heard. The Castro would become the West Coast headquarters of the most deadly epidemic of modern times. Behind the smiling faces and handsome store front windows lurked unsuspecting terror.

The Castro is a district in San Francisco of decorative shops, gourmet restaurants, and crowded pubs. This neighborhood was also once the home of many free-spirited bath houses and private sex clubs. Not unlike DuPont Circle in Washington or Greenwich Village in New York, lesbians and gays revitalized the Castro, refurbishing Victorian homes, opening local theaters, coffee houses, and bookstores. Many of the residents of this district have been acclaimed artists, writers, and educators. There was freedom of self expression. There was a palpable spirit of community. The gay rights movement was forged into the lifestyle of this neighborhood. San Francisco political leaders often lived here. The District and its residents had international prominence. Many health professionals also lived in or frequented the Castro. It seemed a *safe* place to be. Many of its 1979 residents are now dead—AIDS!

In the late 1970's I trained as an Infectious Disease Fellow at the University of California, San Francisco General Hospital. One of my responsibilities was treating patients at the Parasitology Clinic. Parasites connected the third world with the land I then inhabited between two famous bridges. In previous times this clinic treated newly arriving Asian and Hispanic emigrants with a myriad of intestinal worms, shistosomiasis, malaria, and other protozoa. Some patients were American travelers returning from foreign countries with similar infections. Patients who visited this clinic in 1979 were almost entirely young gay men. Most were local San Francisco residents, many living in the Castro and Mission Districts. The majority had not recently traveled outside the country. Many of these men suffered from the malnutrition that frequently accompanies chronic infections of the gastrointestinal tract.

The medical term for the intestinal syndrome seen at this clinic was coined the "Gay Bowel Syndrome." These patients came for treatment of weeping rectal and colon lesions. The necrotic intestinal ulcers harbored parasites, chlamydia, bacteria, and viruses. Patients often had mixed infections, a *venereal smorgasbord.* Doctors such as myself believed we were accurately diagnosing and treating each pathogen. Most patients showed clinical improvement. Repeated infections and relapses were frequent. It never occurred to anyone working in this clinic that passing through the diseased crypts of bowel of these men was a small RNA retrovirus, an unfamiliar pathogen. It was quietly hitchhiking its way into the bloodstream of the accommodating human host. In undisturbed *silence* the virus was sealing its fate into the DNA of our patients and of mankind. Once inside the host, the intruder amplified into billions of viral particles. The quiet invader disseminated throughout the immune system, lungs, gastrointestinal tract, and central nervous system. The unaware host would become ill years later and die as a complication of opportunistic infections and or malignancies. The human death toll would someday reach tens of millions.

The first silent raindrops did not indicate an impending storm. In early 1980 a gay male seen by me at this clinic was admitted to San Francisco General Hospital and rapidly died of an atypical pneumonia and fulminant liver failure. One month later another gay male, admitted through the emergency room, died of a similar pneumonia. They were probably among the earliest casualties of the AIDS epidemic. Four years later the HIVirus would be identified. Like other early cases in Los Angeles and New York, these men never made the AIDS list.

This small RNA virus was kindling disease in scores of unsuspecting gay men by the mid 1970's. It would not be held responsible for years to come. The etiology of AIDS still remains disputed by a few. Humans were selected as a natural host. This intruder came to stay!

By early 1981 unusual cases of Pneumocystis Carinii Pneumonia (PCP) and Kaposi's Sarcoma (KS) were surfacing in gay men in Los Angeles, San Francisco, and New York City. These illnesses were not previously recognized in this patient population. Pneumocystis caused a rare form of pneumonia that was seen in immuno-compromised patients who had renal failure or cancer. KS, an unusual violaceous (raised and purple) tumor seen mostly on the skin, had previously been described in elderly men of Mediterranean extraction. Small population pockets on the African continent were also noted to have this rare skin tumor. The medical community was now witnessing the wrong diseases in the wrong populations in the wrong cities. A medical enigma!

But is the human truly a new host or just an old pal revisited with a vengeance? In millenniums past HIVirus may have surfaced in and out of the old world monkey and human populations. A simian (monkey) retrovirus that possibly mutated has now found permanent residence in the homosapien. Man's intrusion into rain forests and the encroachment on the habitat of other species may have assisted in this selection.

There were no alarm bells then. Now, sixteen years later, millions of lives lost and tens of millions of people targeted to die, and still no alarm bells—still no meaningful public health response. Conservative estimates are that 150–220 Americans acquire HIVirus each day. Worldwide this number is 55 times higher, or 10,000 new cases daily. The virus takes no holidays. There are no coffee breaks. Everyone infected remains contagious for life. There is no cure. The elusive vaccine may never arrive.

The Castro, along with the world, will never be the same.

YOUR DOC CAN'T SAVE YOU

7

I can't save you. No one can save you!
The data is indisputable; nearly everyone HIV-infected will die of AIDS unless other conditions such as heart disease, accidents, or suicide intervene first. Every human being is a susceptible host to this virus.

From San Francisco to Atlanta, from Fire Island to Mykonos, from Port au Prince to Paris, gay communities were taken hostage. By the early 1980's this small invader was causing illness and death to previously healthy gay men. But to the virus there was never predilection to race, gender, socio-economic class, nationality, or sexual preference. Age provided no barrier. Political persuasion did not protect you. Host behavior attracted the attention of this pathogen to the gay population and intravenous drug abusers. This was merely a starting point.

AIDS is now the number one killer of all men in the USA between the ages of 18–44. AIDS is also the leading killer in this nation of men and women *combined* between the ages of 25–45. This is the same disease that was not even imagined just sixteen years ago. It is barely old enough to drive a car.

No human ever infected with HIVirus has been cured—not by natural immunity or medical intervention or luck. Despite anecdotal reports such as the presumed-infected UCLA miracle baby whose HIV antigen test converted back to negative, this phenomenon is extremely rare. Certain newborns who passively acquire maternal antibodies might convert their test back to negative after several months. Those who do are the lucky newborns who, in reality, were never infected in the first place.

AIDS is described as a genome disease. HIVirus incorporates itself directly into the human gene. The virus becomes part of its human victim, quietly replicating within the host's cells. HIV is the blood brother nobody wants!

Once inside the human cell many virons begin a constant replication, others remain dormant. Within a short amount of time one billion new viral particles are produced each day. Eventually over 100 billion viral particles find shelter throughout the body of each infected person. Once a person is HIV-infected, he or she remains infected for life. An individual becomes contagious within days to weeks of initial exposure. The communicable state, like the infected state, is a life-long sentence.

Drugs that demonstrate suppression of this virus in the laboratory *(in vitro)* perform poorly in the patient *(in vivo)*. There is rapid development of resistance to all known available drugs, including the reverse transcriptase inhibitors, tat inhibitors, and protease inhibitors. The virus has a mutation capability that will also hamper the development of future classes of drugs and vaccines. Medical science can save nobody infected yesterday, today, or tomorrow.

The failure of government and private health services to respond to AIDS as a deadly communicable disease, and the absence of personal responsibility, have so far determined the relentless course of this pandemic. Don is one example of how individual responsibility is lacking. He has been my patient for the past two years. His story is not unusual. The path taken by this epidemic includes Don's footprints. He is courteous and friendly. He always keeps his appointments and fits the definition of a "good citizen." To the casual observer he appears socially concerned. He is well educated and actively participates in various AIDS fund-raisers and functions. We have had open discussions about safe sex, but have not always agreed. During the past year Don has visited my office with several episodes of diarrhea. I questioned him about any recent anal sex. He confidently informed me that he was practicing safe anal intercourse with a condom, insertive and receptive. I asked him how many sexual partners he had been with over the past four months. Without a blink he retorted "over ten." I then inquired if he informed any of these partners that he was HIV-positive. Don glibly responded "no," but agreed it might be a good idea in the future. I have no doubt that this polite, attractive, promiscuous gay man, with all his apparent social consciousness, has silently and directly caused others to become infected and die.

Don quietly plays by his own rules. **His unacknowledged actions spread misery and death.** The blood-borne virus possessing this young man could not spread so rapidly without someone's help, unwitting or not. There is no one willing to call Don's behavior criminal. The impact of Don's illness on *himself* is clear. He knows how horrible it is. The impact of Don's illness on others is ignored by Don, health care agencies, and sometimes even by those he infects.

Infection follows every circumstance where HIV-contaminated blood is accidentally transfused. Look-back studies performed by cohort blood banks verify nearly 100% HIV conversion in recipients of infected blood products. The families of hemophiliacs know this scenario all too well. Scientific methodology cannot define percentage risk from each and every sexual or contaminated-needle exposure. Nonetheless, thousands of people are infected by these routes everyday.

People with AIDS brace for repeated opportunistic infections and AIDS-related tumors. The condition is not reversible. The contagious state is never eliminated. Recent data suggests that the greatest period of contagion may actually be during the first several months after exposure, at a time when billions of new viron particles are produced daily. Early on, individuals are without symptoms and rarely aware they are even infected.

The rare long-term survivor is just that, rare and only surviving (never cured). Their survival represents the extreme end of a bell curve. Most long-term survivors still have progressive disease. The long-term survivors followed in my medical practice eventually die of AIDS. The immune system of these patients still demonstrate progressive depletion of CD4 cells (helper T-cells necessary to protect against opportunistic infections). Viral replication continues. The bell always tolls!

The ability to identify any host factors that could alter or prevent infection is crucial to AIDS research. Individuals who might be capable of avoiding the relentless assault on the immune system should be aggressively studied. One small cohort group of possible non-progressors has been identified in New South Wales, Australia. Six individuals who received transfused blood or blood products from the same donor became HIV-positive. During a six to ten year follow-up period, five of the six recipients and the donor have shown little or no progression of disease. Could there be an inherent difference in the immune system of these people? Were they infected by a less virulent (nef gene deficient) strain of the virus? Are they also less contagious? Will they continue to survive?

To better understand the long-term non-progressor, it is essential to know *who* they are and *how* and *when* they became infected. Their clinical course must be followed closely. Uncovering these rare individuals (who are infected but have not developed signs and symptoms of disease) requires a massive HIV screening program. These non-progressors, while feeling well, would not ordinarily be tested or identified. Information gleaned from the non-progressor might eventually shed some light on the development of a vaccine for AIDS.

The virus travels body-to-body. So far there are no surprise insect vectors. Every human being is exposed as a result of the action of someone else. How many readers will someday be infected? A conservative estimate is that 60,000–110,000 Americans became newly infected in 1994. This is roughly the population of the city of Santa Barbara, California. Throughout the entire Vietnam War 65,000 Americans were killed. By the end of 1995 over 329,000 Americans had already died of AIDS. The first round of this epidemic is coming to an end. The human species is taking a pounding and has yet to throw a punch.

When an infected celebrity joins the statistics the demand for a cure intensifies, and once again the roar, "We must educate more!" gets louder. Perverse thinking abounds that if enough famous people get infected *they* will finally do something. The roar always dies down, and the band always plays on.

In the USA we can expect 7 new cases of HIV each hour or 150–220 new cases each day for the coming year. Most, if not all of them (by "them" I mean you and me), will eventually die of AIDS. This virus takes no rest. As the epidemic expands, the number of new cases per hour, per day, per year also steadily increases. The AIDS alarm clock never slows down— it only accelerates. Yet, the ring is barely audible. Some areas in Africa and Asia are currently experiencing exponential growth in infection rate. In Thailand, within a few years, the prostitute infection rate increased from 1% to 40%. In one northern region of Thailand 25% of military recruits tested HIV-positive. Their awaiting spouses are in trouble. The World Health Organization (WHO) predicts that by the year 2000 there may be upwards of 40 to 100 million cases worldwide. Ten million of these cases will be children.

Once you are HIV-infected your status never changes. You remain contagious for life. No one yet has been saved by medical science. Some have been helped, but only temporarily. Your doctor has little to offer. People with AIDS die—you, me, and those we love. AIDS has no cure.

The generation of the HIVs and the HIV-Nots is upon us. The line separating the two is rarely visible. **It can be crossed in only one direction.**

THE OTHER CASTRO

If the Devil doesn't exist, but man has created him,
he has created him in his own image and likeness.

— *Fyodor Dostoyevsky*

8

If it's Cuban, and it's not a cigar, it must be bad. Right? Wrong?

If you want to avoid AIDS, try living in Cuba. The lowest HIV prevalence in the Western hemisphere is in Cuba. The case rate of AIDS in New York City is 15,000 percent higher than that for Cuba.

Communist—yes. Mandatory HIV testing—yes. Protecting its citizens—yes. Rendering care to those infected—yes. Perfect—no. Are we?

Cuba has strict guidelines. If you are infected you are detained, the unspoken word, *quarantine.* The few HIV facilities in Cuba, such as Santiago de las Vegas, are monitored and organized with the assistance of HIV-positive patients and HIV-positive health personnel. Counseling is thorough. Patients are given medical care, provided housing, offered nutritional counseling, and fed as needed up to 6,000 calories per day. They are expected to return to mainstream life. After several months of containment most individuals leave the facility. Detention is longer if an individual's behavior is perceived at risk for spread. 60% of patients reportedly do not want to leave the facility.

It is Cuba's intention to test its entire population. All pregnant women are retested within the first three months of pregnancy. As of June, 1994, four babies have been born HIV-infected in Cuba. Puerto Rico has had over 200 infected babies. The population of Puerto Rico is one third that of Cuba. In the poorest sections of the South Bronx, New York, one in three babies risk being born HIV-infected.

As of 1990, the HIV-positive rate in Cuba was incredibly low: blood donors 0.001%, pregnant women 0.002%, hospital admissions 0.003%, and venereal disease clinics 0.016%. Foreigners and immigrants tested positive at 0.4% and 0.6% respectively. Clearly, Cuba's biggest problem for HIV control is external.

Advantages of Cuba's HIV policy include rapid reduction in the risk of HIV transmission by infected blood products. There is also an opportunity to focus education directly on everyone known to be infected. Unlike residents of the United States, the Cuban population has a very low risk of dying of AIDS.

Government imposed regulation is at the core of Cuba's health policy. By keeping AIDS under control Cuba is able to provide better care for those few infected. Most HIV cases in Cuba are sexual contacts with foreign visitors, or Cubans who did military service in Africa. IV drug abuse is almost nonexistent. Cubans with AIDS don't live in bus stations or on the street. Incidentally, Cuba has a better immunization record and a longer life expectancy for minorities than does the USA. Cuba also has more CT scanners corrected for population than 90% of all other countries in the world.

Is there a precedent for the Cuban model in the United States? AIDS is an infectious, communicable, lethal disease— 20 million people can sadly testify to this. Tuberculosis (TB) sanitariums are set up to offer care for those infected with TB and to protect the public until those patients are rendered non-communicable. Mental health institutions share a similar goal in protecting the public and protecting the patient.

What is the risk of any health facility turning into a jail or concentration camp? It hasn't in Cuba. It hasn't in America.

A greater likelihood would be the creation of segregated communities of uninfected individuals who refuse admission to those who are infected. This is not what I want to see for America. As this epidemic grows more terrifying, even lawyers screaming "discrimination" might abandon ranks and financial gain to join these HIV-negative communities. It is far wiser to apply antilock brakes on this epidemic now. Involve the AIDS community, families, and responsible government to work with a public health service dedicated to prevention. Study the Cuban model. Develop an even better model and be willing to share it with Cuba and the rest of the world. If there is ever a time for global cooperation, it is now.

Placing political ideology aside, Cuba has behaved more responsibly than most other nations in controlling the epidemic within its borders. Health officials there understand universal HIV-surveillance is a mandatory ingredient in performing the public health service that is necessary to protect its citizens. It is more than just a Communist idea; it is a humane gesture to prevent needless suffering and death.

I believe all the above information was worth including in this text. It will give civil libertarians to the radical left and political extremists to the rabid right something in common to be angry about.

TODAY

9

External compulsion can, to a certain extent,
reduce but never cancel the responsibility of the individual.

— *Albert Einstein*

August 31, 1995.
Come spend the morning in my office.

Marcus and I met for the first time today. As he told his story I could think only of my own wife and children. It is so easy not to recognize good luck. In the course of hearing his story I needed to excuse myself. He was beginning to choke on his words. My own eyes were beginning to tear. Over the many years of practicing medicine I had come to believe I had seen or heard of every imaginable tragedy. I have often worried about becoming desensitized to the emotional pain suffered by patients, as can easily happen among health care practitioners. Today, I didn't have that worry.

His story is now part of my life. I will share it just as he related it to me this morning. Eight months ago Marcus was informed that he was HIV-positive. The news came to him straight—not with sympathy, but with rage. It came directly from his wife, "You are infected! You infected me!" They have since separated. He has had to deal with this alone. Two children, ages 3 and 5, have since tested negative, his only blessing.

Before marriage Marcus was promiscuous. This included his involvement with Vicki, who he has

41

since learned is now near death from AIDS back home in Chicago. Shortly following his marriage, an affair with his best friend's wife also occurred. This extramarital activity concluded after the birth of his first child. I have no reason not to accept his story at face value.

When Marcus came to my office this morning he did not appear ill. Although a confessed smoker, he jogs 30 miles per week and is a regular at the gym. He described his wife as being physically well but emotionally distraught. She tested HIV-positive as part of a medical evaluation for an unrelated problem. She took the news of her positive HIV test with utter disbelief. The subsequent CD4 count suggested she had been infected for a number of years. She had no other sexual partners since the beginning of their marriage. Marcus's CD4 count returned lower than hers, indicating that he was probably infected first, and then infected her. Assuming she was infected for five years or longer, each of her children had a 25% to 40% chance of becoming infected as a consequence of pregnancy. Blinded to their illness and fate, no unusual precautions were taken. Both children were endangered by HIVirus through breast feeding.

Marcus notified the woman with whom he had a brief affair shortly after his marriage about his current HIV status. She has since tested HIV-positive, but has had no symptoms. Her husband left her. His HIV status is unknown to Marcus. This woman will no longer speak to Marcus.

I have no medical cure for Marcus. I told him this, but he already knew it. His tragedy cannot be erased. The web of death will continue even after he dies. In the not too distant future his two young children will be without both parents. We will probably try various drug treatments. He will endure physical pain and emotional torment. Someday he will be counted as a statistic by people he will never know.

Marcus's initial physical exam was normal.

I don't know how many other lives are connected to this torn piece of the web. Further tragedy could have been averted if public health had performed universal screening and mandatory contact tracing. By CDC (Federal Centers for Disease Control and Prevention) reported accounts, when intervention is carried out, lives can be saved. A recently reported example is a

Pennsylvania man who notified health authorities of his HIV-positive status. Forty-one previously undiagnosed HIV-positive individuals who had direct contact with him or his partners were tested, counseled, and offered therapy. Studies indicate that direct counseling of HIV-positive patients at the time of diagnosis positively modifies behavior.

The case involving Marcus requires intervention now. Because he does not have clinical AIDS, the health department is unfortunately a nonplayer. Every contact of Marcus should be urgently notified to prevent anyone else from being caught in this web.

Hazel was my second patient this morning. She is 76 years old and was referred for an evaluation of a liver infection. Similar to Marcus, I met her for the first time today. Unlike Marcus, Hazel is HIV-negative. She does *not* have AIDS. It was no coincidence she came to see me today.

While obtaining a family history from her she began to cry. With trembling hands she pulled out of her wallet a tattered memorial news clipping from the local newspaper. She told me what really hurt. Two years ago the 18 year-old granddaughter Hazel raised from birth was tragically killed by a drunk driver on the highway to Santa Barbara. This occurred just a few weeks after her granddaughter's high school graduation. The drunk driver was punished by losing his driver's license for one full year! The medical problem she initially came to see me about was painless in comparison to reliving this tragedy.

I told you Hazel was HIV-negative. What I failed to mention is that Hazel's problem is HIV-related. It is about *personal responsibility*. It is about Mothers (and grandmothers) Against Drunk Driving (MADD). It is about society responding to any reckless behavior that endangers the lives of others.

Phil was the third office patient seen this morning. He is 31 years old, HIV-positive, and recently diagnosed. His monogamous partner of six years continues to refuse HIV testing. Phil has had one serious antibiotic reaction so far. Presently he is tolerating a five drug regimen including antiretrovirals and antibiotic prophylaxis. We discussed adding another drug. Before departing he informed me that a ninth high school buddy was just diagnosed with AIDS in Texas.

The Dow Jones closed up 5.99 points in moderate trading.

WALT WENT NUTS!

The tragedy of life is
what dies inside a man while he lives.
— *Albert Schweitzer*

10

AIDS can make you crazy. Mostly it just saps your senses. Judgment may be impaired. Behavior may be irrational.

You are a pilot, a surgeon, an AIDS educator, a mother. Your mental impairment may affect others: those who trust you, those you love.

AIDS encephalopathy is sometimes, although rarely, the first clinical manifestation of AIDS. Walt complained to me for six weeks that food did not taste the same. Always courteous in my office, he reportedly became involved in a physical altercation with another employee at work, then he beat his own aging parents. This was not the same person I had known for two years. His brain MRI scan confirmed multiple abnormalities. Once described as mild mannered, his family was now afraid of him and found it necessary to confine him to a facility with 24 hour observation that could maintain physical restraints. All treatment failed. Walt died before developing any of the usual opportunistic infections, tumors, blood dyscrasias, or the wasting typical of advancing disease. His clinical course was unusual.

The brain's function can be severely impaired

by a direct, damaging effect of the HIVirus on neuronal tissue or by an associated illness known as Progressive Multifocal Leukoencephalopathy (PML). HIVirus is neurotropic—it directly targets brain tissue.

Then there was you, Arthur. You had us all scared. You spit. You bit. There was never any conversation. Every nurse was afraid to take care of you. No one wanted to feed you. No one wanted to draw your blood. Your assigned doctor asked (begged) me to take over your case. Occasionally a step-daughter showed up. None of us knew you. None of us would. You spit. You bit. That's all you did.

We were your only link to the outside world. All we were told about you from a nursing home was that you once lived in Washington, D.C. It was rumored you were a government man, an economist who worked in the first Reagan Administration. It was said you frequented prostitutes and were bisexual. I had no idea. It was impossible for anyone to obtain a history from you.

Arthur, you died in hard restraints with a CD4 count of 19. None of us ever really knew who you were.

• • • • •

There are opportunistic infections associated with AIDS that have predilection to the brain. Of particular importance is the fungus cryptococcus and the protozoa toxoplasmosis. Patients who are immuno-compromised from AIDS or chemotherapy are prone to these infections. With the growing AIDS epidemic these infections are much more common. If a patient presents with either of these infections, it should be assumed they have AIDS until proven otherwise. These organisms invade brain tissue and impair cerebral function. A patient may otherwise appear physically normal, depending on whether there are other opportunistic infections or tumors. Eventually these infections lead to meningitis or encephalitis and ultimately death. Tuberculosis is frequently seen in AIDS patients and can also invade brain tissue, leading to mental impairment and behavioral disorders.

All these opportunistic central nervous system infections invariably respond poorly to treatment because the underlying immune dysfunction that precipitated infection never improves. The toxic treatment is always lifelong or until the family says "enough." Despite medical intervention, symptoms eventually progress. Initial symptoms, often subtle, include memory loss and apathy. With progressive disease there are extreme headaches, nausea, vomiting, severe confusion and sometimes uncontrolled behavior.

The surest way to warn that these infections may occur is to know who is HIV infected. This would permit families to be aware of what to expect and permit early medical intervention that could ease symptoms and possibly prolong survival. This demands and requires universal HIV antibody screening—for everyone. Hundreds of thousands of people in this country alone could be given early warning and offered earlier intervention for these and other AIDS-related complications. Antibiotic prophylaxis might even prevent the development of these infections. This prophylaxis can only be offered when an HIV infection is identified. Get screened, even if your government doesn't yet have the courage to require it.

THE ENDANGERED GOOD SAMARITAN

11

Only a life lived for others is a life worthwhile.
— Albert Einstein

S he couldn't stop crying into the phone. The call awoke my wife and me. It was the middle of the night. This was my friend, Debbie, a nurse who worked at the hospital. She was now at home.

The call Debbie had just received terrified her; it was from the police.

The prior evening she was returning home from Burbank airport. A motorcyclist directly in front of her was crushed by an oncoming car. The cyclist quickly lost consciousness. In her effort to assist, Debbie was splattered with his blood. A hospital was blocks away. The accident victim survived, partly due to her able assistance. Then the call came from the police. **The police violated the law in warning her.** Thank goodness!

The cyclist was HIV-positive. Hospital personnel recognized him. Her terror began—a three month wait to see if the virus had penetrated her body, a six month wait just to be sure. There would be no sex with her husband or sharing any bodily secretions. The cyclist survived the accident but died of AIDS. Debbie remains uninfected and feels very lucky.

This incident occurred seven years ago. Under the same circumstances would this nurse render first aid today? I do not know. Would you?

Fear is heightened. People think twice before giving mouth-to-mouth resuscitation or assisting with uncontrolled bleeding. One reason—AIDS. An accident victim is 4 to 5 times more likely to be HIV-positive today than eight years ago. Incidentally, so is the Good Samaritan. One reason—AIDS. A lethal epidemic is out of control.

There is another side to this unlucky coin. **The cyclist is your son.** No one comes to his aid. He dies. He is HIV-negative.

ALL THE SURVIVORS ARE DEAD

12

He's the best physician that knows the worthlessness of most medicines.

— *Benjamin Franklin*
(Poor Richard's Almanac, 1773)

*T*he drugs don't work!
Five years ago I received a telephone call from an AIDS patient being cared for elsewhere. He was monitoring a support group attended by one of my patients. The individual who called was emphatic that his own good health was attributed to AZT (zidovudine). With some hostility in his voice he emphasized how improper it was that my patient was no longer on AZT. It didn't matter to this individual that my patient had developed wasting syndrome, did not tolerate the drug, had severe bone marrow depression, and requested that the drug be discontinued. My patient was closely monitored for the development of infection and other complications. Approximately eleven months later my patient died. At his funeral I came to learn that the gentleman who had called criticizing the decision to withhold AZT from my patient had also died of AIDS—on the same day.

The therapeutics directed against the HIVirus is a pharmaceutical Titanic. You never want to be a passenger. Taking the drugs won't save you. Jumping overboard (not taking the drugs) won't help either. Five million people are already dead and another seventeen million people are infected and dying. Twenty-five million more people over the next four years will purchase tickets on this ill-fated cruise. The next generation of fast-track miracle cures are already lining up. They will be blessed by the stockholders, then the AIDS activist groups, and eventually by the Food and Drug Administration. These miracle drugs will certainly have their day in the sun. But as hope begins its ritual peel, the unwelcomed truth will once again be exposed. Drugs cannot save you. Don't get infected. Don't spend the rest of your life praying for new miracles. The Nutcracker is already dancing!

This chapter and the following chapter, "Vaccine Proof," provide a foundation for understanding why **prevention** is so critical. The reader is reminded that as a physician I am convinced that an effective drug regimen that *eliminates* this virus or a vaccine that *prevents* infection will not be discovered in the foreseeable future—a future that may preclude our existence. The issues presented in these two chapters are at times technical and cumbersome, and continue to remain open to debate.

During the past 17 years, as a specialist trained in the practice of infectious diseases, I know of no drug that eradicates any virus causing human infection. Some drugs such as acyclovir (Zovirax) minimally inhibit the shedding of viruses in the herpes class. Amantadine is a drug that might partially inhibit symptoms of Influenza A. But neither of these drugs actually eradicates viruses. Other than a vaccine, there is no drug that effectively eliminates the polio virus, the smallpox virus, or the rabies virus. From the Ebola virus to the common cold virus there are no medicinal cures. Viruses are microbes completely distinct from bacteria, fungi, and protozoa. Antimicrobics kill bacteria and fungi but not viruses. **Does anyone believe the AIDS virus will be the first exception — the first virus ever to be eradicated by an antiviral drug?**

A medical life raft was sighted. Might a derivative of herring sperm (AZT) be the answer to the prayers of so many desperate patients? After the AIDS retrovirus was identified in 1983 by the French, and confirmed in 1984 by the Americans, thousands of compounds were quickly being studied by *in vitro* trials. Many of these drugs had previously been moth-balled for years, having failed to treat other ailments. Feather dusted, and bang, AZT resurfaced as the first panacea for AIDS, a born-again pharmaceutical. This was 1985. Two decades earlier, before any awareness of HIVirus, this drug was employed as a cancer chemotherapeutic agent. It was quickly discarded because of significant toxicity.

AZT is the most widely recognized drug used in combating HIV infection. The mode of action is to inhibit the viral enzyme, reverse transcriptase. This interferes with viral replication. A medical miracle? Hardly! Not even a George Foreman comeback!

Physicians and patients were quick to convince themselves that effective treatment was finally available. Many still cling to this myth. In the early days of AZT therapy, the term "cure" was shared by desperate patients and optimistic academicians. But this life raft had holes. It would rescue no one. Hopes were easily inflated, never the raft.

The HIVirus is resistant to being killed by man's natural immunity. Outside help is needed. Antiretroviral drugs, such as AZT, act by interfering with enzymes necessary for viral amplification. Rapid viral mutation renders these drugs ineffective and viral replication continues. An equally significant problem relates to drug penetration into the specific sites where billions of viral particles reside. To be effective a drug must penetrate directly into the genes of the billions of host cells that shelter this virus. For a drug to be a cure it must reach *every* site of viral replication. The drug must also figure out when the virus is replicating. Dormant viruses that are not replicating are unaffected by treatment. Resting beside human DNA, these latent virons choose a time in the future to unleash and replicate. The virus survives poorly outside the human host but has found a very comfortable home within. This is a very smart virus.

Early studies with AZT were difficult to design. Contrary to how they were published, I believe these studies were never truly double-blinded (neither the patient nor the investigator knows to which drug a patient is assigned). Results from these studies were flawed and prematurely reported. Subsequent studies dispute the original studies. More significantly, the rising death toll disputes any breakthrough. However, I believe that the investigators involved in the first collaborative AIDS Clinical Trial Group studies such as ACTG 016 and ACTG 019 made efforts to remain unbiased. Years later, the benefits of AZT are still being debated; ***the survivors are now dead!***

Different theories have been pondered as to why the conclusions of the initial AZT studies may be inaccurate; why AZT may be a useless drug. The interpretation I offer is given in the context of an Infectious Diseases trained physician, experienced in the care of AIDS patients. Paramount to the understanding of AIDS is the recognition that this syndrome is characterized by an incredibly complex personality. The emotional turmoil accompanying a hopelessly deteriorating physical condition underscores this persona. The social implications are defined by its helpless victims. The numerous direct communications I have had with my patients and their friends and families, the professional contacts I have had with other clinicians, and extensive medical literature review have allowed me to make the following observations. I offer an opinion that remains open to debate.

The early ACTG patients treated with AZT did not represent a cross section of the general population. They did not necessarily represent a cross section of the AIDS population. Almost all of these patients were young to middle-aged white gay men. Very few females were included. Only a few patients acquired illness through blood transfusion or drug addiction. These patients were educated about their illness. Some knew more about AIDS than their doctors. They were acutely aware of the poor prognosis that awaited them. In many circumstances these patients had more access to alternative therapies than their physicians could provide. Some had the networking and determination to obtain these therapies. Many of these men had witnessed the first ripples of this epidemic.

Sexual partners and friends were dropping dead! There was already a sense of hopelessness with treatment. They also perceived (correctly) a government in paralysis and a health care system that was working too slowly. Their disease state would surely progress faster than medical science, and they would be doomed like those before them. Caught in this therapeutic nightmare most of these men sought any treatment that might prolong survival.

AIDS patients begged, prayed, and clawed their way to be kept alive until a cure might be found. Many patients were seen by multiple physicians and at various medical centers. Often these providers, including myself, were totally unaware that these patients were also being treated elsewhere. Total desperation created this "shop-for-a-doc" behavior. Let no therapeutic trial go unnoticed or untried. What was there to lose? Which one of us wouldn't have behaved the same? To this day, AIDS patients attend international AIDS conferences in numbers equal to physicians, research scientists (and, yes, stockbrokers!). There is no medical illness of modern times where patient involvement in drug development and therapeutics has been this inclusive. The AIDS community has been its own strongest advocate.

It is important to appreciate the frame of mind of these patients in 1986 and 1987 who entered the early investigational drug trials. ACTG 002 and ACTG 016 were the earliest collaborative trials designed and reported to be double-blinded, placebo versus AZT. Neither the patient nor the investigator was to know to which arm of the study a subject was assigned. The purpose was to eliminate bias and improve the confidence in results. I believe many of these patients were too smart and too frantic not to know to which treatment arm they were assigned. At this initial point, before the studies even got underway, this indelible flaw of not truly being double-blinded influenced results. This in turn led to erroneous conclusions. I base my belief on the profile of the disease and on the desperation of those being treated. Personal communications I have had with some patients enrolled in these early trials, or with their surviving friends, confirm these suspicions. The percentage of patients who were actually double-blinded is not known. Good intentions don't always lead to good results.

To understand how unblinding influenced the larger ACTG 019 study, it is necessary to scrutinize carefully the different groups. First take the placebo arm. A patient (#1) who had been doing relatively well and had already been taking street-available AZT, and who was then assigned to the placebo group, would likely drop out of the study. The taste of AZT is distinctive. Drug side effects are recognizable. Why would anyone doing well while taking AZT (even if the wellness had nothing to do with the AZT) stop the drug if they were assigned to the placebo arm? They would sooner drop out of the study. The fact that no patient in the study was supposed to be on prior AZT did *not* preclude individuals who were using street-available AZT from signing up anyway. The obvious fact is that many participants were *not naive* to AZT at the time they entered the study. Frightened and intelligent gay men knew how to get AZT through the underground. They understandably did not want to wait for FDA sanctioned trials to begin. Didn't they deserve every therapeutic benefit? They were staring at death. Some patients may have also believed that participation in these drug studies, regardless of infringing upon the double-blinded trial design, would contribute to medical science. So they thought! **Unintentionally, they may have contributed more to medical science fiction.**

The circumstances just described indicate how a healthier subset of patients (#1), who were taking AZT prior to the study, would drop out when assigned to the placebo group. On the other hand, a sicker subset of patients (#2), who had also previously used AZT without apparent benefit, and were then assigned to the placebo arm, might choose to remain in the study. They in fact might have dropped out of the study had they been assigned to AZT, a drug they had already tried and quit on their own. The reader might wonder why these patients (#2) would even bother to involve themselves in this study. It is necessary to appreciate the desperation these people felt (they are now all dead). They sought every opportunity of being followed at one more medical center, by one more group of doctors, maybe smarter than the last group. The price was right; there was no financial burden to participate. They also were afforded the opportunity of close proximity should other future drug investigations become available.

Based on the two types of patients (#1 and #2) described above, I believe the placebo arm of the study selected sicker individuals. These participants were further along in their illness despite the study design that was meant to avoid this bias. Twice as many placebo patients were lost to follow-up evaluation as compared to AZT-treated patients. Curiously, the placebo group also had a 30% higher early drop out rate than the AZT assigned patients. Statistically this should not have occurred unless patients knew to which arm of the trial they were initially assigned.

AZT-treated patients represented the other arm of the study. A patient (#3) already taking street-available AZT, feeling well and assigned to AZT, would likely remain in the study. Now the AZT was provided at no cost. Another patient (#4), one that was not feeling well, was very likely to have already tried street-available AZT. This person, having already experienced AZT with no benefit, if assigned to once again take AZT, was likely to drop out before the study began. The AZT arm of the study was favorably skewed with healthier patients. These patients were also still infected but likely at an earlier stage of disease.

In my opinion the AZT and placebo arms were not created equally. The difference began immediately, on the way to the starting blocks, before the trials actually began. This initial handicapping of the placebo arm explains why early results favored AZT. This also led outside investigators who were independently following results to call off the study early for ethical considerations, falsely believing there was value in AZT. The double-blinded study, that was *never* truly double-blinded, became officially unblinded to the original investigators. AZT would be offered to everyone. *The only thing left blinded was how to correctly interpret the results.*

The AZT arm, on average, was six to nine months later in

disease progression. Since both groups were 100% infected, the AZT arm would shortly catch up with the placebo arm in morbidity and mortality. It is my belief (and I would like to be wrong) that AZT made little or no difference. The *incorrect* message taken from this study, however, was that at last there was effective therapy directed against the HIVirus. Out of this study the "Fool's Gold Standard" of AIDS therapeutics was born. Nearly every subsequent trial of therapy has been compared to AZT. Not surprisingly, the results are impossible to interpret and conflict with one another. Ten years of clinical use have gone by and I honestly don't know whether AZT has minimal benefit, no benefit, or may even be harmful. There have been over 20,000 published articles discussing AZT therapy.

Today there is a better understanding of the natural history of AIDS and the virus-host relationship than there was during the early AZT trials. Remember, this is a newly discovered virus and there have been only a small number of virologists who have ever studied retroviruses. Before this epidemic these viruses were not recognized as significant human pathogens. As a consequence, there were no animal models to study and poor capabilities of culturing this virus. Recent improvements in technology, particularly advances in applying polymerase chain reaction (PCR) and branched DNA testing, now allow monitoring of viral load in blood. This should provide more rapid and objective evaluation of future drug therapies. How scientific investigators will interpret the clinical significance of a change in viral load remains to be sorted out.

The nucleoside antiretrovirals, AZT, DDI , DDC, D4T, 3TC (in order of FDA approval and availability), do not eradicate this virus. They do not cure infection. They may have no direct effect on survival. They will not save a single life.

The use of multiple drugs to inhibit viral replication at different enzymatic sites is at the core of today's clinical investigations. Patients are now offered "alphabet soup" treatment, combining the above drugs with each other or in various combinations with non-nucleoside antiretrovirals such as tat inhibitors or protease inhibitors. Three antiretroviral drugs won't sustain you very long—neither will five or ten. These drugs all have serious side effects. Toxicity is compounded with the addition of each new drug. By adding to drug toxicity, they may actually interfere with the use of other drugs (antibiotics) needed to prevent opportunistic infections. Treatment must be lifelong since the HIVirus is never eradicated. The limited benefit of these drugs is already known by CDC investigators and FDA officials. These are the people who are most aware that antiretroviral drugs will not be the answer for anyone infected. They are the entrusted experts who should be leading the charge for a sound public health policy of prevention—ensuring that AIDS be treated as a communicable disease.

The claim that antiviral drug combinations will revolutionize AIDS therapy is premature. It echoes the past promises of AZT and will spawn similar despair. A brief extension óf survival would come at the expense of major drug toxicity. This is a tough virus, extremely capable of putting down drug rebellions.

A 40 megaton nuclear bomb is about to explode over your neighborhood. An ordinary person, just like yourself, is about to be hurled into the depths of hell from AIDS and its treatment. This person is gearing up for a daily regimen of antiretroviral drugs consisting of 2 epivir tablets, 6 retrovir capsules, and for good measure, 12 ritonavir capsules. Add to the pile 12 ganciclovir capsules if CMV retinitis intervenes (and it eventually will). Alternatively, ganciclovir can be given by intravenous infusions every 12 hours. Since CMV does not go away, the treatment continues until complete blindness or death, usually the latter. Should the toxicity of ganciclovir be intolerable, intravenous foscarnet can be substituted. The yearly cost of this drug is approximately $26,000 (not counting infusion equipment). However, it is extremely doubtful that this person will live out the year.

Most people with AIDS will also be taking double-strength bactrim tablets 3 times a week. If they should develop active pneumocystis, then the dose rapidly escalates to 12 bactrim tablets daily (or intravenous bactrim every 6-8 hours).

Alternatively, intravenous pentamidine, which is difficult to administer and toxic to the kidneys, may be offered. This person can expect to take 5 tablets weekly of zithromax or 1 to 2 tablets daily of biaxin or rifabutin to prevent the atypical mycobacterial infection, MAC (mycobacterium-avium-complex). Should a patient acquire this infection (50% of AIDS patients do), then prepare to take 4 additional drugs, or at least another 10 tablets daily. Since MAC cannot be cured, this treatment is continued indefinitely.

A single diflucan tablet taken 3 times a week might temporarily prevent candidiasis of the mouth, esophagus, or vagina. If cryptococcal meningitis should emerge, then the panic dose of diflucan kicks in—3 to 6 tablets of diflucan daily. At this point intravenous amphotericin B may need to be initiated. This drug frequently causes nausea, vomiting, fever, severe chills, a rapid heart rate, and unstable blood pressure. It also interferes with bone marrow function (which has since been damaged by other drugs). Amphotericin is particularly toxic to the kidneys and sclerosing to veins. These are the veins needed to administer chemotherapy for the various AIDS-related tumors that are likely to develop (if one lives long enough).

Diarrhea can be severe and unrelenting. If the cause is found, such as cryptosporidia, it is usually never successfully treated. This still doesn't prevent one from trying at least several different therapies. Struggling to swallow so many pills is never easy, especially when the mouth is covered with the sores of oral herpes (stomatitis). Five acyclovir capsules taken daily might alleviate this condition, but only temporarily, since herpes always returns in the immuno-compromised AIDS patient.

If this person is still physically capable of complying with treatment, by now he or she will likely be consuming 40 or more pills each day (and spending a great deal of time kneeling over toilet bowls). Next, here come the drugs to stimulate the appetite—4 pills daily of megace or marinol. If there is any resulting depression, this can be managed with a choice of antidepressants. By now, well-meaning friends and relatives will be recommending a handful of antioxidants and herbs.

In the event of itching or a drug-related rash, the physician, who is teetering on AIDS burn-out, will be left to guess which of 17 different drugs to discontinue. But don't feel sorry for the "doc." He or she can always walk away from this chemical battlefield—the patient cannot!

As the body continues to waste, the HIV-patient might be offered (if the HMO insurance allows) intravenous hyperalimentation with lipids and amino acids. Certain to be anemic, epogen injections will also be considered. Experimental human growth hormone injections could be made available, but at an annual cost to the patient of $60,000. Like other therapies, this cost will be prorated by the week or the month. Patients on last ditch treatment rarely survive much longer. When the central venous line becomes infected, the time-honored antibiotics will be called upon to rescue whatever is left.

It is entirely possible there will *never* be any effective antiviral therapy to cure AIDS. The "V" in HIV stands for virus. There is no drug that eradicates any virus. The demands to "release the drugs" and "AIDS treatment now" clamored for by concerned activists will never be satisfied. The antiretroviral drugs already released are nearly worthless. They certainly do not render a cure. Included on the new drug list are the protease inhibitors: saquinavir, ritonavir, and indinavir. The media hype and the Wall Street thirst for this new class of drugs is enormous, but the therapeutic benefit is already recognized to be limited. While these drugs may demonstrate a favorable drop in viral load, they will not rid anyone's body of this virus. Any benefits will likely be short lived. The euphoria currently being generated will dissipate along with those unfulfilled drug promises of yesterday. Every dollar in the world thrown at the problem won't insure a cure. Changing presidents won't insure a cure. An AIDS March to the Moon won't save lives!

Most patients treated with antiretrovirals have already died, including the self-proclaimed cured. Others are gravely ill and will soon die. HIVirus takes its time, but its ultimate devastation makes even the Ebola virus look wimpish. Once HIV-infected, don't hope you are the *one* in 100,000,000 who will escape. There are better lotteries. Don't get infected in the first place. Treatment is dismal. Not a single person infected with HIVirus has had this virus eradicated from his or her body, not by AZT or any other conventional or unconventional therapy. Not even close! Never! Nunca! The message must be prevention.

The greatest single benefit of antiretroviral drugs is *not* about how they impair the HIVirus. The benefit is that such treatment leads to closer supervision by health care providers. This improved monitoring results in earlier treatment and prevention of the opportunistic infections that kill patients. As a consequence of better treatment of AIDS-related opportunistic infections, survival is extended. The patient remains HIV-infected and HIV-contagious, but lives longer.

Only a better understanding of the basic science of the immune system could ultimately save lives. Recently the Office of AIDS Research (OAR) at the National Institutes of Health pushed for changes in scientific priority. The emphasis shifted in support of unsolicited, investigator-initiated research as opposed to pharmaceutical-originated (profit-oriented studies). Resources are strained. To continue to spend tens of millions of dollars determining whether AZT barely works, hardly works, or doesn't work at all is unethical. Science must open new frontiers. To continue to remodel the bedroom while the kitchen is on fire is insane. Don't be part of the inferno. Don't get infected!

The Australian chestnut bark is now replacing the Chinese cucumber of the witches brew therapies. In desperation new experimentation with alternative and underground treatments is constantly being tried. These include ozone, hypothermia, hyperthermia, and hundreds of herbs and botanicals. Patients travel to Calistoga, California, to cleanse their bowels with mineral water colonics. A patient of mine attempted to align the electrons of her body with the North Pole using a homemade electromagnetic chair. For ten weeks she swore to its benefit. She died shortly thereafter.

Because of the potential for litigation, the patient relying on unconventional treatment is usually the experimenter as well as the experimental subject. As hopeless as many of these underground remedies appear, they may be no better or worse than "The Real McCoy," AZT. The outcome is always the same. These patients don't survive and the treatments are shortly discarded. Unless there is obvious and immediate harm, it is difficult to dissuade anyone from using alternative therapy. If one is dying and all conventional therapeutic modalities have failed, what is to be lost?

Those who network in the AIDS underground monitor nonprescribed therapies. To their credit, they are usually quick to point out adverse effects. This network has also coalesced much of the AIDS community, helping to channel patients into social services that provide the more basic needs of food and shelter. While the "Drug-of-the-Month-Club" may never come up with a magic bullet, it has been able to sustain hope and provide compassion where conventionally practiced medicine has failed.

Testimonial cures attributed to all these therapies, conventional and cult, are ultimately buried along with the patient. The AIDS quilt will soon cover the face of the earth. Each patch now serves as a warning flag that prevention is our best and only hope. There may never be a cure.

In the time span of the next ten days the world will witness enough new cases of HIV-infection to pack a football stadium as large as the Rose Bowl. During this same time period we will be lucky to have added one new AIDS scientist. Research funds are scarce. The limits placed on science and health services are no match for the limitless number of future patients.

How long do we plan to wait for a miracle drug?

VACCINE PROOF?

Too bad we just can't sue the virus
and immunize ourselves against lawyers!
— Pam Savitch, RN

13

Not everyone can be as lucky as a Gambian prostitute!

Man will never set foot on the surface of the sun. Man cannot reverse the axial rotation of the earth. Similarly, an effective AIDS vaccine may be beyond man's reach.

Smallpox epidemics once ravaged the world with death. In 1796 Edward Jenner demonstrated the utility of smallpox immunization when he inoculated eight year-old James Phipps with cowpox fluid. This infected material was obtained from a sore on the hand of dairy maid Sarah Nelmes. Jenner was an astute bird watcher. His observations as an ornithologist undoubtedly assisted him in observing that milkmaids with cowpox (vaccinia) were cross-protected against smallpox. On the seventh day after James Phipps was inoculated with cowpox he complained of discomfort in his arm pit. On the ninth day the child developed chills and a fever. The following day he was perfectly well. Five weeks later he was inoculated with material taken from a smallpox pustule. Small punctures were made on the boy's arm. The contaminated smallpox fluid was carefully inserted. No disease followed. Several months afterwards James was again inoculated with smallpox fluid. Again, no illness followed. The child was successfully immunized. Jenner's experimentation antedated the germ theory of disease. His brilliance gained him admission to the Royal Society of London. Viruses were not discovered until over a century later.

Smallpox, which used to sweep the globe with massive epidemics, has been completely eliminated by immunization. Fatal outbreaks of polio, diphtheria, measles, and other infectious diseases have been dramatically reduced in size and frequency by active immunization programs. Vaccines have saved millions of lives and prevented social disruptions. Today, the Edward Jenners of science and their bold, brilliant actions are handcuffed. No doubt present-day American lawyers would hang Jenner, the Royal Society of London, and most of England on the spot.

I attended a national AIDS forum in early 1985. This was approximately one year after the discovery of the AIDS retrovirus. Optimism abounded that an effective vaccine would soon be available, but probably not until the early 1990's. That timetable seemed much too slow for those of us who were watching the death toll mount. And now, the hour that was to bear fruit has even passed—there is no AIDS vaccine. Instead we have come to realize that this smart virus came well prepared. This genetic blood brother resides comfortably alongside human DNA. It elicits no protective immune response from the infected human host. It pays no rent.

A vaccine stimulates the body's immune system to produce antibodies against infectious agents. Immunization prevents illness or ameliorates the severity of symptoms from future exposure to the live, natural microbe. Most vaccines that are utilized against viruses and bacteria are live-attenuated or killed micro-organisms.

The ideal immune response of a vaccine is to produce antibodies that mimic a natural infection. At a future time of exposure the body's immune surveillance would recognize the infectious agent and martial a heightened antibody response to the microbe. This rapid immune response of neutralizing antibodies aborts serious infection. An individual who becomes infected without prior vaccination, and who then survives the illness, will usually develop protective antibodies against future infection with the same organism. This happens with mumps, measles, and chickenpox. It is generally accepted that natural infection produces the greatest and most sustaining antibody response.

The enigmatic HIVirus is distinguished by its failure to elicit a protective neutralizing antibody response following initial exposure. As though regarded as family, the human immuno-surveillance does not recognize this virus as foe. Instead it incorporates this virus into the human genome. Not behaving like a stranger, one might wonder how many times this virus may have paid a visit to the human species in millenniums past. The antibodies that are measured for HIV testing do not inactivate the virus. As a consequence of this failure to control viral amplification, there is rapid spread to more host cells and other body tissues. The virus remains alive and well and always prepared to find a new host.

Essentially all humans serve as a natural host to this virus. To date, any genetic protection is sketchy. The CCR-5 mutant gene demonstrated in 1% of certain European populations is claimed to be associated with a lower risk of sexual spread of HIV. One small group of high risk HIV-negative Gambian prostitutes are reported to exhibit a cytotoxic T-lymphocyte immune response (cellular immunity) following repeated HIV exposures. Validating this or any discovery of "natural protection" is crucial in the design of a future vaccine. For the vast majority of the world's population there are no recognized protective barriers beyond the intact skin and mucous membranes. I believe that further investigation will reveal that no group is protected and that the apparent luck of the Gambian prostitute will run out.

The task to develop an AIDS vaccine with fragments of a dead virus, or a whole live-attenuated virus, or even a genetically engineered virus is likely impossible. A vaccine generally does not elicit a stronger immune response (protection) than the natural infection. Unfortunately for humankind, the natural infection with HIV does not neutralize this virus; it is unlikely that any type vaccine would do better. An effective AIDS vaccine would be a remarkable pioneering achievement in immunotherapy. The hidden doors to a better understanding of the immune system have yet to be discovered, let alone opened. Enmeshed in the riddle of AIDS immunotherapy may also reside unanswered questions about cancer.

Animal models are difficult to study with the HIVirus because no other species is as accommodating a host as man. Most large primates such as baboons seem impervious to the AIDS-causing virus, just as humans are impervious to the simian virus that causes SAIDS (an illness similar to AIDS found in the monkey population). Chimpanzees and gibbons are endangered species that are not widely used as animal models. Recently it was discovered that the Pigtail Macaque, another primate cousin, was also vulnerable to becoming infected with HIVirus. This primate can become infected but it does not become ill. Live vaccines that have been used in all of these animal models have met with disappointing results and may prove to have no human application.

Of major concern is the fear that a live HIV vaccine carries the risk of causing AIDS. This could result as a consequence of viral mutation of the vaccine strain by continued human passages and replications. This is the fear of all live vaccines. The potential to immunize and thereby infect the entire population with a weakened strain of HIVirus, that can itself lead to AIDS, is clearly not the answer.

The immune system is under constant invasion by this virus, particularly the T4 lymphocytes of the reticuloendothelial system (lymph nodes). The lungs, gastrointestinal tract, and the central nervous system are also targeted. Billions of new HIVirons are replicating throughout the body within weeks of initial exposure. Some people experience a mild flu-like illness. Most people have no clue that they have been infected. The virus remains dormant in the genes of many host cells. In other cells it is amplifying and preparing to attach to new, uninfected CD4 cell wall receptors. The recent capability of measuring viral load suggests that the initial wave of viral amplification is so great that the host is immediately contagious.

Most bodily tissues eventually become engulfed. The infectious state will continue until the death of the host, often many years later. When a steady state is achieved it is estimated that 100 million to 1 billion new viral particles are produced daily in each infected person. During this ongoing replication, the human host, in declining health, still fails to elicit any significant neutralizing antibody. The expectation that a vaccine could eliminate this virus when years of exposure to the natural infection could not produce effective neutralizing antibodies is wishful speculation. Attempting to develop a vaccine to accomplish what the natural infection fails to accomplish is novel.

If ever a miracle vaccine were to be developed against the HIVirus, could it keep up with the rapid mutation of this virus? The organism is constantly altered during its many lifecycles. The virus with which one is initially infected changes its genetic composition with ongoing replication. No two AIDS viruses remain genetically identical, and this ongoing mutation or change significantly complicates the development of a vaccine.

Don't be misled into thinking that the blood of a monkey in the wild will save anyone. Preliminary studies with passive immunization (giving immune globulin with high concentration of HIV antibody) have not been rewarding. This treatment has not saved a single life. It is extremely unlikely that anti-serum, derived from dying AIDS patients, will benefit another dying AIDS patient. It certainly did not protect the donor. Why would it protect the recipient? These antibodies simply do not effectively neutralize the virus. Passive immunity is no cure and will unlikely prolong survival.

What about xenografting (replacing human tissue with the tissue of another primate such as baboon bone marrow)? The assumption is that these foreign cells are resistant to the HIVirus. However, it is very unlikely that the baboon marrow cells will reproduce and not be rejected by the human body. Furthermore, the billions of live virons already outside the bone marrow of the recipient are not affected by a donor transplant. How many baboons would have to be sacrificed to treat 20,000,000 people and save no one? Will we replace other body parts with baboon parts? Will there be baboon farms? Wouldn't it be better for humans to behave responsibly, by stopping the spread of infection within its own population, and thereby spare the baboon?!

A strong argument for a comprehensive universal HIV screening program is to identify the possible existence of a very small subset of the population that develops antibodies but avoids illness and a decline of the immune system as measured by the CD4 count. Might these rare individuals, who are referred to as non-progressors, have developed cellular immunity? The improved ability to measure viral load will also determine whether long-term non-progressors even exist. Universal screening is necessary to identify such a group. These people would be without symptoms and unlikely to be tested or otherwise identified. The benefits of universal testing must be extended into avenues of vaccine research.

Many vaccine investigations have been canceled because of poor results and legal snarls. Other vaccine research programs have been eliminated because of insufficient funds. Most countries conduct no scientific vaccine research. This is occurring at a time when AIDS will soon be the leading cause of death in the world.

As demonstrated with smallpox, an effective vaccine would clearly be the best means to eradicate AIDS. Our present understanding of immunology is not adequate to develop an AIDS vaccine. Furthermore, no vaccine would likely benefit the tens of millions already infected. In 20 to 40 years from now that number could exceed 1 billion people. It is quite possible mankind is light years away from ever realizing an AIDS vaccine with only calendar years to survive. This virus has set the immunologic clock back to the time period of Edward Jenner.

Less than 7% of American doctors routinely provide care for people with AIDS. Research scientists are an even rarer breed. Whenever I lecture at a high school or college and ask the question, "Who here might consider AIDS research as part of their career?" there is near silence, even astonishment. For each scientist currently being trained to do AIDS research, our finest universities are graduating over 900 attorneys. Brain power is dangerously being wasted. The Dream Team of Jenner, Pasteur, and Salk has been replaced by Cochran, Bailey, and Shapiro.

ABOUT TO EXPLODE

14

No matter what we look at,
the first step toward the highest human ability is,
I think, the effort to look at it correctly.

— Shin'ichi Suzuki

I hated to throw things out. I promised to finally clean out the garage. It had been years. My wife deserved a place to park her car.

A dust-covered box caught my eye. About to be tossed was a slide carousel dated 1982. I decided to take a peek.

The carousel contained old slides from the first lecture I had ever given on AIDS. My talk was at a medical grand rounds conference for a local community hospital. I held a slide up to the direct sunlight shining in from the open garage door.

312 cases in the USA! History was in my hands. The fate of my species was unfolding, slide after slide:

Gay white men ... GRID (Gay Related Immune Deficiency) ... San Francisco, New York, Los Angeles, Paris, Rome ... Many cases in Central Africa ... Haitian connection ... Brussels, Belgium—origin Zaire ... Possible infectious agent ... Amylnitrate, sexual enhancer, suspect ... Kaposi's sarcoma ... Pneumocystis carinii pneumonia ... Cryptococcal meningitis ... Toxoplasmosis of the central nervous system ... Oral thrush ... Bath house closures ... Patient "Zero," Gaeten Dugas, French Canadian airline steward ... No treatment available ...

In late 1982, standing at the podium, I would never have predicted that within the next fourteen years the world would witness tens of millions of people dying from this strange new disease, and it would spread unchecked, person-to-person. The generation of "free love" would come to an end. It could cost you your life. Sexual expression of love could be turned into an act of death, even murder.

By 1996 half of the *new* cases in America would be heterosexual. The American epidemic would become Africanized (the majority of cases being heterosexual). By the end of this century half the new cases would be *female*. At last, equal rights!

EARLY INTERVENTION
For Treatment And Prevention

15

It is better to be looked over than overlooked.
— Mae West

If you are HIV infected you must know. It is not going away. Seize any opportunity that might prolong the quality of your life. **Care enough to not infect and kill someone else.**

There are many compelling reasons to initiate universal screening. Topping the list must be protection of those uninfected. This is the only group that has a chance to survive this epidemic. To control transmission it is necessary to know who is infected. This applies to every contagious disease. Sexual preference of those afflicted does not alter this basic principle. Early intervention by public health authorities can only be effective if not thwarted by those committed to treat AIDS as a civil rights issue. While we protest against *not* having a miracle cure, we ignore the obvious. Let Public Health perform public health!

The USA is estimated to have 90,000 new HIV conversions during the next year. Without intervention by public health services this number will increase with each successive year. None of these new converters will be aware they are in the early disease period unless they are HIV tested. This large group will further spread

71

infection, resulting in an acceleration of newly infected cases. Each new converter can expect to eventually die of AIDS.

Medical intervention should be considered as soon as possible after infection. This includes treatment, counseling, and contact tracing. To accomplish this requires a universal screening program that encompasses everyone and is nondiscriminatory. Such a program will provide better control of the spread of this virus by identifying newly infected cases shortly after exposure. Partner notification is essential. Risk behavior must be modified and, when necessary, monitored. Essentially, this is the application of public health procedure as applied to all other contagious diseases. AIDS, unquestionably the most lethal contagion, deserves this same effort.

Early identification offers the opportunity to evaluate the benefit of treatment at the first stages of infection. Only universal screening could identify the untold number of unsuspecting Americans and millions of people worldwide who are infected and contagious, and could be offered early medical intervention. Improved technology offers the opportunity to monitor viral load and assist in evaluating new therapies.

The majority of people infected today have not yet been identified. It is guaranteed they will eventually surface, but only too late. To offer early medical care it is necessary for patients who are without symptoms to first be identified. Some investigators believe that any benefit of antiretrovirals (therapy directed specifically against the HIVirus) in prolonging life would most likely occur by combining antiretroviral drugs and treating at the *earliest* possible stage of infection. This remains to be seen. This "sooner the better camp" points out that billions of viral particles are present within weeks after initial exposure. This is also the time when the host immune system is still intact. Maintaining the integrity of the immune system and decreasing the viral burden at the earliest stages of infection is crucial. This is at least the theoretical argument behind early medical intervention. It is not known if early treatment might diminish the contagious state. Treatment at the later stages of disease, when an AIDS diagnosis is finally made, offers at best only marginal benefit. By some accounts, treatment with antiretrovirals at advanced stage of disease may actually be harmful. Man's medicine cabinet is void of drugs that eradicate any virus. The expectation that an antiretroviral drug will be discovered that kills the AIDS retrovirus, similar to how antibiotics kill bacteria, will never be fulfilled. We should at least try to maximize any benefits from the drugs that are available.

A recent multi-center study, ACTG 076, concluded that initiating AZT treatment to infected pregnant mothers along with follow-up treatment of newborns decreased by 68% the incidence of HIV conversion of newborns. Will this stand up to the scrutiny of further investigation? If these results are accurate this study would represent one of the few instances where an antiviral effect was demonstrated by any drug. The CDC was finally prompted to recommend all pregnant women be HIV tested. About time!

Risk factors that lead to infection and have previously not been recognized could be identified by universal screening. Current assumptions about safe sex and the role of saliva and other bodily secretions must be challenged scientifically. AIDS education that is fueled by political rhetoric, overshadowing the need for scientific discovery, is unsatisfactory and misleading. HIV screening would help clean up AIDS education.

Public health measures have failed miserably to contain AIDS. They have strayed from the tradition of protecting the public's health. Why the complete breakdown for an incurable disease? Why is there still argument about mandatory reporting, mandatory contact tracing, and even mandatory testing? **Where is the mandate to save lives?** This is not radical, rabid, or right-winged medical thinking. This is just correct medical thinking.

Only full-blown cases of AIDS are reported to most county health departments. Just being HIV-positive doesn't count. Spreading the virus doesn't seem to count either. Reports are used for calculating statistics as to age, gender, race, type of exposure, and so on. The statistics are then passed on to

State health departments for their scrutiny and reporting. Eventually, agencies such as the CDC publish national figures. Broad recommendations, with no teeth, accompany these reports. The World Health Organization (WHO) also keeps its own scoreboard.

Periodically there are cries of alarm and calls for more education when a shocking statistic is released. Unfortunately, they result in a continuation of the policies that are already in place—those that are not working and don't include intervention. The CDC will quietly recommend a new group for voluntary screening, such as pregnant women, always testing the political waters first.

A Princeton University thesis points out behavioral changes that accompany a knowledge of one's HIV status. Retrospective studies demonstrate the use of testing and counseling to favorably modify behavior. Comprehensive testing along with public health service intervention to guarantee safe behavior is required to temper the pace of this epidemic. One prospective analysis looking at a worst case scenario, which includes no testing, counseling, or behavior modification predicts a minimum 70% population drop-off by the middle of the 21st century. This is compared with present population figures. The social upheaval would be so enormous as to be incalculable. Only draconian governmental intervention would be left to cope with the tide of death. HIVirus has no plan to leave on its own accord. Why are we not instituting humane and effective measures needed now?

The very difficult and most important part of AIDS education, frequently avoided and painful, now begins. *A lifelong and personal commitment of every infected individual is required to control this epidemic.* Every HIV-infected individual must be identified and carefully counseled. These people are contagious for life, regardless of symptoms. Customary behavior could be deadly. It is also the responsibility of those uninfected to remain uninfected. The human species has been changed by this virus!

A comprehensive screening of all women of childbearing age must be initiated. This is to alert health authorities and also these women of their HIV status. No one should be denied therapy when a benefit can be demonstrated. 50% of babies born HIV-positive are delivered from mothers who do not know their own HIV-positive status—many thinking they are not at high risk. 7,000 HIV-infected women delivered babies in the United States in 1993. 32% of those newborns became infected.

An argument is made by civil rights loyalists that a mother of an infected child should not be automatically informed of her own child's HIV-positive status. It is maintained that this is an infringement on the privacy rights of the mother—that by informing the mother of her baby's status it would infringe on the mother's right not to know her own status. We have become so entangled in laws that we are willing to compromise health to the extreme. I am not so sure that if we stumbled upon a miracle cure for AIDS we would still have the common sense to use it!

Antibiotics that are administered to prevent opportunistic infections prolong the lives of patients with HIV. A large number of people who do not know they are HIV-infected have already progressed to a state of severe depletion of their immunity, yet many of them have not manifested symptoms of disease. Consequently, they are not identified as being HIV-infected. Therefore, they are not offered the timely prophylactic antibiotics that could prevent or at least delay opportunistic infections and improve the quality of their lives. To properly identify this large group of unsuspecting people, universal screening is mandatory.

All women of childbearing age should be HIV tested. *All civil libertarians who disagree with this should also be tested!* Every partner of women of childbearing age should likewise be tested. What is wrong with protecting women and their newborns from a deadly disease? In fact, the fastest growing group of new HIV infections is heterosexual females. The best guarantee to protect the newborn is to have a mother who is not infected. By 1994 New York City alone had 30,000 AIDS orphans. Next door, in New Jersey, there were an additional 10,000 AIDS orphans. Many of these young children, orphaned by AIDS, will themselves develop AIDS and die, motherless. The best guarantee of having a mother who is not infected is to be sure she is not inseminated by someone who is infected. *We all need to be tested.* The process of testing, counseling, and intervention is enormous. But it is worth it.

Universal screening means that everyone be tested: male, female, gay, straight, old, young, newborn, Black, Caucasian, Asian, Hispanic, doctor, and patient (if you are left out, you need testing too). EVERYONE! The World Health Organization and the United Nations should be actively involved in assisting all nations in this endeavor. This is the challenge to control AIDS. This is the requirement to preserve humanity.

NO GOOD DEED GOES UNPUNISHED

The salvation of this human world lies nowhere else than in the human heart, in the human power to reflect, in human meekness, and in human responsibility.

— Vaclav Havel,
President of Czechoslovakia
(Address joint meeting of US Congress)

16

I've known Matt for seven years. He is a hospital social worker. On weekends he volunteers at a community homeless shelter. He is like gold. I've never seen him anxious before. He asked if we could talk.

Matt's story is as follows. He and his wife had temporarily cared for a three year-old child. The child, a nephew, lived at their home for two months while the child's mother was hospitalized. The illness was not disclosed, but they were led to believe it had something to do with her liver. Out of concern for the child's welfare they volunteered, along with other family members, to help.

During the time they cared for this child no unusual precautions were taken for nose bleeds, scraped knees, and the like. Tooth brushes were shared with their own children. The little boy seemed to have frequent sniffles but otherwise seemed healthy.

After good-byes and thank-yous they found out that the mother had AIDS and that the little boy was HIV-positive. The diagnosis had been known since birth. Matt's family was shocked. He was visibly upset sharing this with me. Could the lives of his wife and children have been unnecessarily jeopardized because they did not take proper precautions? I reassured him that the risk of HIV transmission was low but I could not tell him how low. I was not there for each cut and scratch. He wanted to be absolutely sure there was no spread of infection. It was decided that all family members be HIV antibody screened. The tests would be repeated in 3 to 4 months. During that period of time he and his wife could choose to abstain completely from sex because of the remote possibility that either of them might have become accidentally infected. Condom protection was not good enough. They were advised to share no bodily secretions. They would pray.

Matt's concern did not end there. The infected child never received medical attention or drug prophylaxis to prevent opportunistic infections. There was never any inquiry made by any public health officials. There was no established physician to call in case of problems. Matt's home is still open to this child.

• • • • •

Let me now tell Stephen's story. I knew him less than 48 hours before he died. By the time we first met he was so confused that I don't think he ever knew who I was.

Stephen presented to his primary care physician one week earlier with headaches. There were no signs of wasting or chronic disease. A spinal tap was performed and a diagnosis of cryptococcal meningitis was made. His HIV test returned positive. His CD4 count was very low. Stephen rapidly succumbed despite heroic efforts with therapy. His case was unusual, with a very rapid mental decline in an otherwise healthy appearing man.

At his death bed his parents first learned of their son's HIV diagnosis. During the week after his death, Stephen's grieving father contacted me. He wanted to share a concern. Did I think his son might have previously known of his HIV status? I had no answer. There was something else he needed to tell me. A year earlier his son was assaulted while parked in his car. Gay bashing was the explanation given. The car windows were shattered. Stephen was badly cut and required medical attention. The car was towed to his Dad's house and the two of them cleaned up the glass and blood with _bare hands._

I counseled him about HIV testing. "Stephen was always such a good son," he lamented, "Why didn't he tell me?"

HEADS IN CEMENT

Don't worry; the universe is expanding,
so it doesn't matter anyway.
— *Salik Shah*
(1976-1994)

17

We are blind to what is happening.

Six o'clock p.m. headline news: "New Glove Evidence Introduced Today ... Senator Packwood Declined To Comment On ... Nine Thousand Marchers Join In Annual AIDS Walk To Fundraise Money For ... Two NATO Warplanes Were Fired Upon Over Bosnia According To ..."

On the sofa a three day-old newspaper shows a front page picture of Bob Hattoy, captured under an article titled, "White House AIDS Activist Falls Into Political Exile." In this article, President Clinton, who calls this disease his "passion", is accused of abandoning the cause, neglect, and hot air. So, what else happened today?

150 to 220 Americans became HIV-infected today. One teenager became infected every hour. This is repeated each day of the week, each week of the year, and year after year. The number of new cases each day will gradually increase with time. Not a single person who has ever been infected has been cured. AIDS could even kill Superman.

AIDS is a painful journey. HIV is universally fatal. There is complete failure of drugs to eradicate this virus (and all other viruses). A miracle vaccine is not projected. Society certainly has the right to expect that stringent public health measures are implemented to control this epidemic. Halting transmission is imperative to save lives. To date we have not erected any public health policies that will prevent transmission. Do we lack courage, compassion, common sense, or all of the above?

Just who had discovered the RNA retrovirus that presumably causes AIDS? The summer of 1984 witnessed a medical scandal simmering across the Atlantic. The Pasteur Institute in Paris and the National Institutes of Health (NIH) in Bethesda, Maryland were at odds. At stake was ego, fame, ethics, patent rights, and of course, lots of money. The two contesting parties were Dr. Luc Montagnier in Paris and Dr. Robert Gallo in Maryland. The French insisted the virus was given to the Americans the previous year for investigation. The Americans initially denied the claim. Future medical cooperation was in jeopardy. Despite the controversy, great strides were made in discovering this virus. But then what?

Ten years later, 1994. Americans continue to believe tax dollars contribute to public safety. Then, a stinging revelation occurs on tax day, April 15, 1994. The Centers for Disease Control and Prevention (CDC), the definitive government source for health information, publishes alarming self-critical findings issued by the National Academy of Science. The Academy reports that the CDC is in trouble—that the CDC can't do its job. The Emperor of Health publicly declares his own nakedness. Is anyone listening?

The frightening truth regarding public health failure is announced in three reports issued by the National Academy of Science. These reports point out the inability of the United States public health system and health professionals to confront emerging infectious diseases. The Academy reveals that the capability of State public health laboratories to support the surveillance and control of infectious diseases has diminished. Despite the emergence of contagious diseases, control efforts have actually declined over the past decade. The National Academy of Science warns that the public health services in this nation are in disarray!

The CDC repeatedly claims in its self-published Morbidity and Mortality Weekly Reports (MMWR) that the way to prevent sexual transmission of HIV infection and other sexually transmitted diseases (STDS) is to avoid sexual intercourse with an infected partner. The agency encourages the widespread availability of testing, claiming it is essential to identify asymptomatically infected persons. These are our top dogs preaching the obvious. Now they must insist on the obvious. Now they must lead. Now it is time for all of us to practice the obvious.

Knowledge of HIV seropositivity has been associated with subsequent decreases in risk behavior. The CDC's own opinion is that HIV counseling is more likely to be effective if accompanied by HIV testing. There is almost unanimous agreement that universal screening accompanied by mandatory reporting and counseling, and focused partner notification, would help abate human losses.

Funding for the CDC is inadequate. The morale at the CDC is low, witnessed by an alarmingly high personnel turnover. The agency now does little more than decree general recommendations to combat disease. Epidemiologists both within the CDC and other health care agencies know full well that AIDS is out of control. The practice of epidemiology needs resuscitation.

The public health system in America is beyond the need of upgrading—it warrants a complete overhaul. It's too late for a coronary artery bypass—it is time for a heart transplant. The public health measures that are necessary to control the AIDS epidemic will be formidable to implement and painful for many. Standing on the educational soapbox and hoping for responsible behavior is passive suicide. This virus will not change its behavior; it is up to us to change ours.

The time has come and gone for mere soft recommendations. Entrusted public health officials must be mandated the authority to fulfill the obligation of protecting public safety. Many public health officials have carefully played the game of political correctness. This has secured their jobs.

It has also assured the AIDS virus a permanent home in the human species.

Teach the truth! It is criminal to spread this virus! It is criminal for health care agencies to watch this happen and not respond! Millions of people around the world will become infected this year alone and will eventually succumb to AIDS. Every imaginable public health policy to curb transmission and stop the carnage must be considered. Additionally, there can never be separate political consideration for sexual preference when a deadly new pathogen threatens our entire species. The penalty for being late is being paid for today in horrendous human suffering.

HIVirus is *highly* contagious by intimate contact. While "intimate" contact is a relative term, susceptible to personal interpretation, it occurs frequently enough to have fostered the spread of the most serious plague of modern times. Each person is infected by their own actions or by the behavior of someone else. Any doubt about this being a highly communicable disease should be put to rest. Those who simply refuse to accept its contagious prowess must explain themselves to the millions of people who are already dead, and to the countless others who are infected and ill-prepared to die.

This virus ignores all of our therapies and all of our policies. It does not care if its human host is politically right or politically left, gay or straight. Over 22 million people have already joined the global AIDS death march. Five million of us have already been stilled and silenced.

By choosing not to provide public health safeguards now, many more lives will be sacrificed. Future generations will find it far more difficult to do what is appropriate and necessary to contain this virus. More people will be infected tomorrow than today, and every public health measure will be more challenging to implement. The quality of care available to each patient will diminish as thinning resources are shared among more and more infected people.

The AIDS epidemic shows no signs of natural burnout. Might this virus continue to spread until there is no one left to infect? While science deliberates over whether antiretroviral drugs fail or fail miserably, and while the public anxiously awaits a vaccine that is "in the mail" but might never be delivered, more people are getting infected. *Preventing transmission* remains the only option to combat AIDS. How long will this truth be ignored?

IRON CURTAIN DOWN
AIDS CURTAIN UP

I'm an atheist, thank God!
— *Michael McLaughlin*
(Cate School, Class of 1995)

18

The Cold War is Dead. Cold Reality is Alive. "Don't get infected. They don't want you." China, Taiwan, Japan, Singapore, Albania, Russia, Ukraine, Cuba, Afghanistan, Saudi Arabia, Iran, Lebanon, Kuwait, etc.

Russia is harsh in its response to AIDS. More specifically, "non-Communist" Russia is harsh in its response to AIDS. Hundreds of HIV-positive foreigners have been deported over the past eight years. The spread of AIDS is associated with infected travelers. The former Communist nation has passed into law that no visitor, student, journalist, or business traveler is allowed to stay longer than three months without verification of an HIV test. This has incited an expected clamor from AIDS activists groups and certain proclaimed AIDS experts. An expert is someone who can cure the disease, not someone who can render an educated opinion. There are no experts!

The Health Ministry in Russia reports 154 people dying of AIDS and 967 others known to be HIV-infected. Activists claim these numbers are much higher, perhaps as much as ten times— all the more reason for health officials in Russia to focus on prevention. In the USA the number of active AIDS cases has surpassed 519,000 and the number of HIV infections possibly exceeds 2,500,000. The same activists claim these numbers are also low. Considering a population size comparable to the USA, the Russians have been spared so far.

Now the Russians are criticized for not adopting the two-pronged, Americanized version of AIDS prevention: First, educate those uninfected on how HIVirus is believed to spread. Second, teach responsible behavior to those already HIV-infected (even though you don't even know who most of them are), and then hope they behave responsibly.

The scoreboard indicates how poorly AIDS education is controlling this epidemic in the United States and in most of Europe. The broader lesson, signed into law by Boris Yeltsin in the Fall of 1995, tells the world the Russian people cannot afford AIDS. Their social structure is already in turmoil. They admit to not having the medical capabilities to handle this disease. They plan to attempt prevention on every front, including their borders.

Russian health officials correctly believe that only HIV-positives can spread this disease. HIV transmission is more readily spread in those countries where there are no controls. An alternative for health officials in Russia would be to require that all foreigners be HIV tested. Those testing positive must be regularly followed by a health official during their stay. Smacks of the old KGB! HIV-positives don't want to give up their privacy or sexual freedoms to government control. After all, someone else infected them. Activists are infuriated over the decision by the Health and Foreign Ministry officials in Russia. The Russian people, *free* to speak at last, so far have shown little objection.

The once rich United States now owes the world 5.1 trillion dollars. That is twelve zeros. And it's growing. This is $800,000,000 worth of interest *daily*. POOF! Does this sound like the winner of a Cold War? This country can no longer take care of its disenfranchised, its homeless, its sick. When the cumulative cases of AIDS double in the next four to five years, what resources will be left to take care of cancer, heart disease, and all the new cases of AIDS? The United States is facing a health care crisis today. Tomorrow will be chaos. We must adopt a stringent model for AIDS prevention for the sake of those not yet infected, who will likely receive worse medical care than those already infected. Our energy would be better spent fixing things at home than pressuring the Russians to adopt our *failed model* of AIDS prevention.

The Russian government is doing what it can to protect the Russian people—to keep them alive. If it means restricting the rights and privacy of visitors, they believe it is a fair trade off.

The world must relate as a community to control the AIDS pandemic. Universal testing, which is necessary, must be that—universal! Anyone testing HIV-positive needs close supervision by officials in the country in which they reside. Every nation has a responsibility to the world community to control AIDS. Every nation has an obligation to its own people to prevent the spread of a deadly pathogen through its own population. The global challenge to stay alive is enormous.

INVOLUNTARY MANSLAUGHTER

No man can put a chain about the ankle of
his fellow man without at last finding the other end
fastened about his own neck.
— *Frederick Douglas*
(Washington, D.C., 1883)

19

It did not take very long. The world's blood and plasma were being poisoned. By 1982 hemophiliacs (individuals genetically deficient in producing blood clotting factors) were manifesting symptoms of the strange disease that was killing gay men. This signal was loud and clear. It was *blood-borne*. No malice. No premeditation. Within eight years 50-70% of the hemophiliac population would be wiped out as the result of receiving contaminated blood products. This would happen to my friend, Bonnie Frasier's, three hemophiliac sons.

I returned Jorge's call. He is my first cousin by marriage, a good man, and a lawyer to boot. Jorge asked if I would see his aunt. Juanita was 74 years old. She had lost 30 lbs. over the past four months. She had progressive weakness and intermittent fevers. She was told she might have cancer. She lived in another part of the state. Jorge would bring her to see me.

Juanita frequently traveled to her native home of Peru to visit family. She also worked as a Red Cross volunteer. Ten years prior her husband underwent coronary artery bypass graft (CABG) surgery. He had been transfused blood during surgery. Five years later he developed persistent headaches. An MRI scan of his brain revealed multiple lesions. Believed to be beyond benefit of a biopsy procedure, the family was told that his brain abnormalities were probably metastatic tumors (cancer spread from a site elsewhere). He died within weeks.

Jorge's aunt showed severe signs of muscle wasting. She was weak and short of breath. My first response was to ask her to open her mouth. Her tongue and oral cavity were covered with the white thrush of monilia (fungus). She had AIDS. In retrospect, her husband also had AIDS. His brain tumors were probably toxoplasmosis. His bypass surgery had killed them both.

Elizabeth Glaser acquired AIDS as a complication of a blood transfusion at Cedars Sinai Hospital, Los Angeles, in 1981. She subsequently founded the National Pediatric AIDS Foundation after she learned that her two children had acquired the disease, the first through breast feeding, the second through pregnancy. She pioneered for AIDS awareness and led an effort to rid the stigma associated with having AIDS. Elizabeth and her first child have since died. Political activist Paul Gann met a similar fate following a blood transfusion. So did tennis star Arthur Ashe. These people are well remembered.

There is also 83 year-old Thelma White. I took care of her six years ago when she was diagnosed with Alzheimer's Disease. It just so happens she also had two large brain lesions on a CT scan. Her HIV test returned positive. She was also transfused during elective hysterectomy surgery in 1984. There are many Thelma Whites to remember.

EDUCATE THE EDUCATORS

20

Save your mistakes for bad movies, final exams, and stock market investments. They give you a second chance. AIDS does not. An educational blunder about AIDS transmission magnifies into thousands of lost lives. Never forget HIVirus is lethal. No doctor, drug, or vaccine will save you. Always err on the safe side. Always!

How we educate about AIDS may be dangerously flawed. What we educate about AIDS may be dangerously inaccurate. The science behind AIDS is incomplete. The politics surrounding AIDS education is derailing prevention.

Certain AIDS educators claim that this disease is *not* highly contagious. This is supported by the belief that casual contact does not spread the virus, that intimate exposure to blood and bodily secretions is required. While this may be true, it is not reassuring. Explain this minimally contagious concept to the tens of millions of people who have already become infected by person-to-person spread. Perhaps we need to redefine intimate exposure and recognize that its natural frequency is extremely common. AIDS may be communicable enough to eradicate our species. To teach that AIDS is not very contagious is *dead wrong!*

Intimate contact is here to stay—to the very end. It occurs every split second somewhere on the planet. Saliva and genital secretions are commonly shared, some might suggest causally. Intimacy is normal, healthy behavior. Its frequency varies with culture and personality. Let's accept intimate contact as something that will not and should not vanish. It is necessary for procreation.

HIVirus is transmitted in the arena of intimacy, including normal sexual behavior. Normal is defined by the participants, not by the "Church Lady." Let's just keep it safe. One analytic study demonstrated a 69% reduction in HIV transmission with the use of condoms. 99.9% is not good enough! **Safe means knowing the HIV status of your partner, not just using a condom.** Only the virus knows where casual contact ends and intimate contact begins. Humans have the difficult task of defining this boundary.

The gay community, a leading proponent group for education, cannot contain the epidemic within its own ranks. This tragedy is played out every day. Read the obituaries! A front page article in the *Los Angeles Times* discusses young gay men straying from safe sex. This article cites that half of these young men, ages 15 to 22, are engaging in high risk, unprotected sex. 10% of this very young group are *already* HIV-positive. How many more of these kids will be infected after another five years of high risk behavior? Concern is also raised, in light of new statistics, that many older gay men are ignoring the safe sex message. There is no group in America which has personally witnessed as much death from AIDS as gay men. There is also no group more educated about AIDS.

Education is not curbing the AIDS epidemic. Surveys on university campuses throughout the United States point out that the majority of students are well educated on how AIDS is transmitted. Most don't feel personally vulnerable. The majority have unprotected sex. If they were to be tested, counseled, informed of their own status and had an open and honest relationship with their partner, then other educational tools would likely hit home. Merely waiting for the result of ones own HIV test can be very sobering.

The benefit of education is clearly limited if our goal is to save lives. If education could miraculously cut the transmission rate by 50%, and we were down to only 5,000 new cases per day worldwide instead of 10,000, or if in the year 2000 we only saw 37 million cases instead of the projected 40–100 million, would this be cause for celebration?

Some psychologists support the wisdom of focusing more attention on HIV-negative men. They challenge the claim that this kind of attention is divisive and stigmatizing, robbing HIV-positive men of attention and resources. I believe HIV-negative individuals (regardless of sexual preference) must have knowledge of the HIV status of their partner before plunging into any educated adventure.

Standing alone, HIV education is not succeeding. Why? Are we incapable of learning? Is AIDS education repetitive motion without substance? Might AIDS education have more impact if it included AIDS testing and the reality that a positive test is a death sentence? Blind counseling does not stick! Relying solely on education may in fact be fueling this epidemic because it is replacing other sound public health practices. AIDS education must hammer home the importance of adhering to the principles of epidemiology that apply to all communicable diseases. The incurable AIDS virus is *no* exception. AIDS education has failed miserably to make this point. *Giving educational lip service to testing and partner notification is like placing the kiss of death on lovemaking.*

You have a better chance of winning the state lotto 3 times in a row than being cured of AIDS. AIDS education must make it unmistakably clear that never getting infected in the first place is what counts. There will be no monkey antiserum, magic bullet, or spontaneous remission. Education must emphasize responsibility; that once infected there is no jeopardizing anyone else's life under any circumstance. **Blatant irresponsible behavior is blatant murder.** Whatever lifestyle adjustments are necessary, make them!

A person who is HIV-infected should *never* engage in

contact sex or share bodily secretions with anyone who is uninfected. This necessitates all partners knowing whether or not he/he, he/she, she/she or the entire group is infected. This requires everybody being tested. Testing requires repeating on a reasonable schedule. Universal screening is necessary to combat this epidemic, whether or not believed or taught by your AIDS educator. This process will be cumbersome, inconvenient and *life saving.* Your privacy may be encroached upon. This will also be exceedingly easy and relatively painless to accept when compared to the unsuccessful treatment of millions of Americans with AIDS, possibly including yourself, in the years to come.

According to George Washington University sociologist Amitai Etzioni, promoter of communitarian thought, HIV control must include majoritarian inroads upon personal freedom. "Half of the story we tell is about rights, and we put them first. When we as a nation mindlessly multiply rights and ignore the responsibilities that go with them, then we actually undermine the rights."

I have never met anyone with AIDS who felt the pleasure that led to their infection was worth it. The suffering is horrible. Every person I have ever treated with AIDS would have gladly accepted any public health measures that might have averted their tragedy. The best AIDS educators are those individuals suffering and dying with this infection.

Today we are witness to the consequence of isolated, incomplete, and sometimes inaccurate AIDS education. Despite our current efforts of education, the world sees eight new cases every minute. In America it is estimated there is at least one new HIV case every seven minutes. This clock never stops. Heterosexuals now comprise almost half of all new cases in America. The world's gay population has already been decimated. HIVirus has saturated the gay male population as much as 50% in some inner-cities.

The American and European hemophiliac populations have not been spared. The story hasn't been any better in Japan. Hemophiliacs represent three-fourths of all cases of AIDS in Japan. Of the approximately 5,000 Japanese hemophiliacs, more than 1,800 were infected with HIV through contaminated blood-clotting agents *imported from the United States.* Despite warnings of possible contamination, there was intentional disregard for HIV screening of blood products by Japanese health officials. One Japanese woman shared her experience. She contracted AIDS from her husband, who was a hemophiliac and died of AIDS. His treating physician did not even reveal to them that her husband was infected. The Japanese people hold their state guilty for allowing the spread of this deadly infection.

In the American teenage population the rate of HIVirus infection is reported to be doubling every 4 months. Catastrophic! In a national school-based youth risk behavior survey, 54.2% of students in grades 9-12 reported having had sexual intercourse. 19% had 4 or more partners, 50-60% did not use condoms. Most teenagers are well informed about HIV transmission. Information is not deterring the spread of this virus. Well informed people are dying of AIDS! Included in the ranks are many AIDS educators.

The AIDS virus is transmitted through shared contaminated needles, sexual contact, sperm and tissue donation, transfusion of contaminated blood products, and from mother to newborn. Read the above sentence 100 times. Now you are AIDS-educated. Do you feel safer? Are you 100 times more likely to change your behavior? I vividly recall as a school child the disciplinary action of certain teachers when my class was unruly. This consisted of repeatedly writing the same sentence on a piece of paper or at the chalk board, sometimes for an hour. Today I can only remember the disciplinary action, not what we wrote. The educational value was lost.

Retrospective studies in the USA and Canada observe a low rate of transmission of HIVirus to nonsexual household members. Many of the families evaluated were of hemophiliac patients. The HIV status of the infected member was clear to everyone in the family. Appropriate precautions were taken. The low rate of transmission under these circumstances is reassuring and underscores the importance of knowing who is HIV-positive. What is not available are careful studies of families where the status is not known and precautions are not observed. However, there is an increasing number of documented AIDS cases that have been reported among siblings and other household members. These were felt to be mostly bite-related, although a shared toothbrush was also implicated.

What is protected intercourse? What is safe sex? What is the value of your life? How do you value someone else's life? **How strong is the commitment not to kill someone else?** That someone may be a person you love. Reality is harsh. One of my patients who is HIV-positive refrains from any sexual activity with his uninfected wife. No bodily secretions are shared. He will take no further chances. He reminds himself that she is the mother of their child. His child will soon be without a father.

There are a number of published reviews regarding safe sex and various methods of protected intercourse between infected and uninfected partners. These articles essentially outline the rules of Russian roulette, which now has application to latex, vinyl and lubricants. *There is no safe contact sex between an infected and uninfected individual.*

Don't bet your life (or someone else's life) on a condom, damper, or lubricating disinfectant! The mechanics involved in the sexual transmission of HIV are not fully defined. Specific HIV receptor cells on vaginal and rectal mucosa permit viral attachment. These viral receptors are also present in the mouth. T4 receptor sites exist in lymphoid tissue throughout the body. Abrasions on the mucosal walls lining the vagina and rectum, caused by sexual trauma, allow this virus to penetrate into the blood stream. The virus also invades through skin tears and abrasions inside the mouth. Associated venereal infections such as herpes, chancroid, or chlamydia create a friable mucosa. This also assists the entrance of HIVirus. Any sexually transmitted disease (STD) should alert health care providers of the heightened risk for AIDS. The World Health Organization now estimates 360,000,000 annual cases of STDS. Every STD demands an HIV test and a negative result should be followed by repeat screening in 3 to 6 months.

How contagious are nonblood secretions? What is the incidence of blood contamination in saliva and semen? HIVirus can be cultured from almost every nonblood secretion and bodily tissue. The significance of the viral concentration in these other fluids is not well understood. Enzymes in saliva inhibit the virus, but its true protective capabilities leave question. Partial inhibition is totally inadequate when a single viron may be all that is necessary to initiate infection. Millions of viral particles exist in a single drop of infected blood. An Italian study found 91% of saliva specimens to be contaminated with blood after passionate kissing. Blood contamination in saliva is 100% with proper tooth brushing. How soon does blood clear from saliva? When do the gum abrasions completely seal off? Each tear in the mouth is a source of blood seepage as well as a portal of entry for this virus.

Some biological truth is difficult to accept. Some biological truth is painful to swallow. *Some biological truth is fatal to ignore.* HIVirus is in saliva. HIVirus is in salivary tissue. HIVirus is certainly in blood in tremendous concentrations. Saliva is further contaminated with blood as a consequence of tooth brushing as well as of passionate kissing. Both leave abrasions in the mouth. Hepatitis B can be transmitted by saliva and kissing. So can many other viruses. *Until proven otherwise,* so can HIVirus (I am willing to take the heat for such a bold statement about a lethal disease). Somewhere between 0.7%–2% of the U.S. population is HIV-positive. Passionate kissing is not safe without knowing the HIV status of your partner. It is easy to ignore certain biological principles when they do not fit our desires or suit our behavior.

The natural history of other blood-borne viruses cannot be ignored. Hepatitis B is endemic throughout Africa and Asia. Neonatal and sexual transmission of Hepatitis B is common. Blood product contamination, IV drug abuse, and fecal-oral spread are also frequently recognized. Hepatitis A, Hepatitis C, Epstein-Barr Virus (EBV) and Cytomegalovirus (CMV) all have either fecal-oral or salivary modes of transmission. EBV is the virus that causes the classic "kissing disease" known as mononucleosis. All of these viruses are larger in size than HIVirus and have no trouble making their way into the blood stream. These analogies for transmission may not be identical to HIVirus, but the red flag shouldn't be ignored.

Is the "dirty deed" required? Sexual transmission of AIDS might encompass an oral-oral or genital-oral route, not necessarily transmitted only through penile-vaginal or penile-rectal intercourse. To the conventional AIDS educator this smacks of heresy. The reality is, we don't know the extent of other risk factors. Acquiring AIDS from oral sex is recognized. Transmission from semen through abrasions in the mouth has been documented. A 1993 Surgeon General's report to the American public on HIV infection emphasized "getting semen, vaginal secretions, or blood from an infected person into your mouth puts you at risk of HIV infection. The risk of getting HIV from oral sex is not as high as from anal or vaginal sex, but there is risk. Sores or cuts anywhere in your mouth would make oral sex even more risky." What the Surgeon General neglected to emphasize is the obvious—the importance of knowing if your partner is HIV infected!

The response to the Surgeon General's warnings that came from the Office of AIDS of the California Department of Health Services was an eight-pronged set of guidelines. They advised about lubricants and coverings for a partner's genitals. They cautioned against sharp objects such as fingernails, jewelry, dental braces, and chipped teeth. Left off this "list to save lives" during oral sex (fallatio, cunnilingus, anilingus), was the most important warning—never have oral sex with anyone who is HIV-positive or whose HIV status you do not know! What or whom are these AIDS educators afraid of? These entrusted officials are conditioned to be politically cautious when they should be clinically cautious. What they should be teaching is that it is imperative to know the HIV status of anyone you share any secretions with—if you don't know, don't do it!

The animal model of simian AIDS is not perfect, but it is the best we have. In a recently reported study in the journal, *Science,* researchers were able to infect six out of seven rhesus monkeys with the simian AIDS virus by gently placing the virus on the back of their tongues. None of the monkeys in this study had any oral lesions or cuts. Even more startling, the researchers discovered that the concentration of virus needed to infect the monkeys was only one six-thousandth of what was necessary to infect them rectally.

The risk of contaminated saliva is understated. French kissing or passionate kissing is associated with a continuous sharing of saliva. When was the last dental flossing or brushing—5 minutes ago, 30 minutes ago? A peck on the cheek and a French kiss may not be the same in the eyes of the virus. No prospective study could ethically be done that exposed HIV-negative volunteers to the constant infusion of saliva from an HIV-positive donor. No one would volunteer. No one should volunteer. Those who deny the possible risk of saliva are unlikely to come up to bat themselves and participate in any such study. The political climate influencing AIDS education encourages, "what we don't know is probably safe." **AIDS educators should not be willing to bet anyone's life on what we don't know.** AIDS education may not always be safe!

This virus enters your body without a passport or a greencard. No one should give permission. There are no early warning symptoms. The easiest way to confirm infection is to test for antibody. AIDS education must encourage the use of every tool, including universal testing, to prevent the spread of infection. We teach traffic safety to save lives. We enact laws to enforce traffic safety. AIDS education requires the same support to save lives.

The most AIDS-educated group of patients I treat is gay men. Despite education this population continues to be saturated with HIVirus. This is also true for the new generation of young gays. The future will continue to see young gay men with AIDS. The future will continue to see middle-aged gay men with AIDS. If we continue the *same education,* the future might be without any *old* gay men!

IN MEMORY OF ALL THE BOBS

21

I will never forget the shock of seeing Bob walk into my office. I can still see the sadness worn on his face. Not you! That was all I could think. Certain moments in life leave a permanent imprint.

Those of us old enough remember exactly what we were doing and how we felt when President John Kennedy was shot. I was in the tenth grade. It was third period. We were dissecting a frog in biology class. Another student from another class ran into the room with the unbelievable news. That afternoon I sat with friends at a drug store counter eating french fries, drinking a cherry coke, and listening to adults talk and weep.

I can also never forget the moment in 1969 when Neil Armstrong stepped onto the moon. I was lying on a gray, itchy rug, next to my cousin, focused on the television screen.

There was another moment, much more recent. October 6, 1995, 10:03 a.m., West Coast time. The entire world was glued to television and radio. The O.J. Simpson Verdict was announced. At the time I was talking with a 19 year-old AIDS patient in an exam room. This was Sean's first visit to see me. He was not promiscuous by history. There was no intravenous drug abuse. He was tested at the insistence of his mother. His CD4 count was high, indicating he was only recently infected. Years from now he will become ill. One can only hope he infects no one else. There is no jury to convince here.

I'll never forget Bob. I first met him a year prior while renting a tuxedo for Tim's wedding. Bob was the sales clerk. He was a gentleman. I never knew his last name until he later became a patient. His primary physician had referred him to me because of an unresolving pneumonia and an AIDS diagnosis. He was added to the day's schedule. What must Bob have been thinking when he saw me?

Tim is somewhere between my best friend and an adopted older son. He is the ultimate package, a big brother to my younger children and a baby-sitter. Tim lived with us for three years while he attended college. On the deck in back of the house, in front of the crashing surf, we would sometimes talk all night. It's funny how Tim was always too cold and I was always too warm. These were the few moments we both shared with the ancients. Under an umbrella of stars it was easy to convince ourselves just how unimportant and fleeting life's problems really were. We determined our own lives to be merely a bleep in time and space. We had Washington, D.C., figured out. Tim referred to this period of man's history as the "Frustration Period." We also selected our own all-time NBA basketball team. We knew everything that was wrong with the world. Lawyers were given no mercy. We both made predictions about the futures of my children, Jessica, Rhett and Teague, since he knew them as well as I did. We loved each other's company and still do.

In 1987 Tim got married. I was proud to be part of the wedding ceremony. I have never been thrilled with wearing a tuxedo, but for Tim's sake I could suffer one afternoon in a monkey suit.

Everyone met at J.C. Penney to get fitted for Tim's big day. For Tim, a college student, the tuxedo ordeal was a financial stretch. Up walked Bob, the sales clerk. He was dark-complected. a small man in physical size but a giant in courtesy. We were impressed by his kindness, patience, and concern that all go well at Tim's wedding. He must have come from a generation when gas station attendants checked your car's oil level and washed your windows so your journey would be safer. Bob was so endearing that he became Tim's last invited wedding guest. I did not see Bob again until the day he walked into my office, one year later, frail and shivering.

Bob survived fifteen miserable and depressed months. He thanked me after each visit. The few holidays he had left to share with anyone never went without a small, thoughtful gift for my staff and me.

There is a Bob living next door to you. He is at your church. He is in your family.

YOUR WORST TOOTHACHE

When a dentist makes an extraction
you hope he pulls the tooth,
the whole tooth, and nothing but the tooth.
— Anonymous

22

D o you feel lucky?
You work in West Hollywood. You are HIV-
negative. You need oral surgery. The oral surgeon
in your building will fit you into today's schedule.
He is HIV-positive. 30% of the patients he treats
are HIV-positive. It's time to spin.

There have been a number of outbreaks of
hepatitis B virus (HBV) associated with dental
procedures. There are probably many other
sporadic cases whose origin was at the site of a
dental instrument and went unrecorded or
unrecognized. Blood and saliva contamination
occurs between dental patients and sometimes
directly from the dental worker.

It is impossible to adequately autoclave all
dental instruments. Heavy equipment is
stationary and not transportable for sterilization.
Sterile technique can turn sloppy. The amount
of care taken by the operator and technical failure
are factors. There is not adequate control for
aerosolized or misted blood-containing particles.

The routes of transmission of hepatitis B are
similar to those of HIVirus under the
circumstances that include sexual spread,

shared-contaminated needles, transfusions, and neonatal exposures. Dental workers have one of the highest rates of hepatitis B exposure. It would be wise to assume HIVirus poses a risk of spread through dental procedures similar to hepatitis B.

On August 21, 1987, the CDC published recommendations for prevention of HIV transmission in health-care settings. Pertaining to precautions for dentistry it was stated, "Blood, saliva and gingival fluid from *all* dental patients should be considered infective." Interestingly, nine years have elapsed and the CDC has never warned of the dangers associated with passionate kissing and swapping of blood-contaminated saliva. **Why not?**

The transmission of hepatitis B or hepatitis C complicating hemodialysis or other medical procedures where there is any failure of technique, breakdown of hygiene, or mere accident will likely apply to HIVirus. They are all blood-borne diseases. Before the availability of the hepatitis B vaccine, 50-60% of chronic hemodialysis patients contracted hepatitis B. This was primarily associated with the breakdown of environmental technique in infection control. Slightly lower numbers are associated with hepatitis C. HIV transmission in hemodialysis units has already occurred. In Columbia, 22% of patients in a single dialysis unit converted their HIV status as a complication of inadequate disinfection technique. The risk is real but the extent of danger cannot be measured without HIV screening. Any person who is identified as being HIV-positive should not share any dialysis equipment with any other person who is HIV-negative! Dialysis patients should be repeatedly screened for HIV because symptoms of infection may not manifest for years.

Patient-to-patient transmission of HIV at private surgical centers has also been described. In New South Wales, Australia, five surgical patients reportedly acquired AIDS from a single source. All underwent minor surgical procedures on the same day in the same operating suite. The surgeon was HIV-negative. Improper hygiene could not be identified but was believed to have resulted in patient-to-patient transmission.

In two major US cities, one being the nation's capital, it was recently reported that improper technique occurred during work site vaccination programs. This resulted in HIV and hepatitis screening of all those participating. Most accidents of this kind go unnoticed and unreported.

Three patients at separate locations undergoing nuclear medicine procedures were inadvertently injected with blood or other contaminates from patients infected with HIV. Two of these patients became HIV-infected and the status of the third is unknown. These are certainly aberrant occurrences, but they cannot be ignored. In view of the fact that HIV is steadily increasing in the general population, this kind of transmission will become more frequent.

The actual number of dental workers who are presently infected with HIVirus is not known. Testing is arbitrary. There is no reporting. Only those testing negative would likely report their status anyway. HIV-surveillance studies are voluntary, and those dentists who know they are positive are not likely to participate. A dental worker identified as HIV-positive is usually advised to follow the guidelines of the State Dental Association. Their strongest recommendation is to follow strict hygienic technique and avoid dangerous procedures. The criteria for danger is left to the discretion of the infected practitioner.

In one community of which I have personal knowledge, a particular dental worker performing invasive procedures was found to be HIV-positive. The status surfaced as a consequence of HIV screening as part of an insurance physical. Local public health officials were alerted because of possible public endangerment. They chose not to intervene. Legal risk factors weighed heavier than health concerns. This cowardly decision was made with trepidation. Silence followed. No one felt comfortable. I privately asked other health officials if they would allow this dental worker to treat them. With one exception there was a resounding "no." When the single exception was questioned further, it was acknowledged that this dental worker would not be allowed to treat this public health official's child (but it was okay to treat your child!).

The final unofficial decision made by public health officials was to permit this dental worker to practice anonymously without any patient awareness or choice.

Does HIV transmission occur as a complication of dentistry? The American Dental Association (ADA) suggests that dental-related transmission of HIV is an unusual occurrence. They do not know the true risks—neither do I. Only by mandatory HIV screening and reporting, and by careful analysis of all other risk factors, can a meaningful attempt at answering this question be made. Since there is no universal screening, any inadvertent exposure is unlikely to be uncovered. In the situation of hepatitis B virus (HBV), there is an incubation period of 3 to 6 weeks before symptoms develop. Infected individuals can be traced to a common source, especially in a community wide outbreak. The source can be a food handler, a contaminated water supply, and in some circumstances even a dental office.

HIVirus is far more capable of avoiding detection than HBV. The initial HIV infection is usually silent. Many years can transpire between exposure and the time symptoms develop. Without a program of universal HIV screening it is extremely unlikely that any person infected at a dental office, who has no significant initial symptoms, would ever associate the original source. The first signs of illness may not occur until many years later (also many years after potentially spreading this virus to unsuspecting others). By the time AIDS is actually recognized the infected individual will be anguishing. _How_ and _when_ could this have happened!? The real question is _why_ did anyone let this happen. Patient "x", identified 9 years later, may have already infected multiple sexual partners. None of them may have visited the dental facility where the outbreak originated. It is possible that an entire network of cases, numbering in the hundreds, could erupt in this manner. Without universal surveillance of the asymptomatic population, the common source might never be identified. Most of the infected people would likely not even know each other. Each infected branch of this "tree of death" would be unaware of the other dying branches.

The case of dentist David J. Acer gained national attention in July of 1990 when the US Centers for Disease Control and the Florida Department of Health and Rehabilitative Services reported the first identifiable outbreak of AIDS from a common dental source. Six cases were traced to Dr. Acer's office in Port St. Lucie, Florida. The outbreak intrigued the media. Mike Wallace of *Sixty Minutes* and other television news magazines dissected every detail with the assistance of private investigators. National and local health officials conducted their own investigations. Rumors included deliberate murder and sexual abuse. The more benign accusations included inadvertent exposures and poor office hygiene. All the infections had a nearly identical RNA composition to that of Dr. Acer. Supposedly none of the patients were previously acquainted. Furthermore, none of the patients were able to recall any injury to the dentist that might have exposed them to his blood.

The most unusual aspect of this outbreak was the mere fact it was recognized. The first identified infected individual was 21 year-old Kimberly Bergalis. She became ill within a relatively brief time after exposure. She recalled hearing of Dr. Acer's illness. A careful search eliminated all other risk factors except for visits to his office. With Dr. Acer's *permission* a look-back program was set up by health officials to screen other patients rendered care by him. **For a brief moment the practice of epidemiology was revitalized.** The tracing identified five additional cases that demonstrated genetic similarity with Dr. Acer's retrovirus. In total 0.5% of those patients treated by Dr. Acer became infected. Interestingly, in the process of doing the appropriate screening, several unrelated cases (different RNA sequencing) were also uncovered.

To date the actual mode of transmission in the Acer outbreak remains a sad and unnecessary mystery. Improper hygiene or possible sociopathic behavior on the part of the dentist remains unknown. To avoid possible self-incrimination it is believed Dr. Acer was advised to avoid full cooperation and disclosure. Dr. Acer died of AIDS with the full tragedy of this story untold. Some argue that this outbreak was a fluke event. The true fluke event was that the HIVirus in Kimberly Bergalis took an unusually virulent course and her symptoms surfaced early. This may be the single factor that alerted her and health officers to the connection with Dr. Acer. Most of the time this virus is more careful, taking cover longer. It is time for us to be more careful!

The most obvious risk factor to control is the HIV status of the health care provider. This is also the risk factor health officers dare not touch. There is no risk of acquiring infection without exposure to an infected individual, even from an accidental blood exposure. The prevalence of HIV in the health care provider is directly proportional to the prevalence in the general population. The risks associated with dentistry, however small or difficult to identify, will continue to increase as the epidemic spreads. Thirty years ago the population was HIV-free. There was no dental risk to patients regardless of technique, hygiene, or who previously occupied the dental chair. As the general population became more HIV-saturated, so have dental providers. Today there are also geographic risk factors. The root canal performed in Greenwich Village, New York, may carry a greater risk of HIV exposure than the same procedure performed in Thermopolis, Wyoming. If there is any improper hygiene, you'll have wished you could see the Grand Tetons and not the Statue of Liberty from the window facing your dentist's suite.

Gums are vascular and bleed easily. Dental procedures abrade the gums. The purpose of a dental drill is to drill and the intent of a dental pic is to pick. Mucous membranes are a protective barrier to infection just as the skin is a first line of defense. Dentists and hygienists work in areas of the oral cavity where visibility is poor. There is exposure to sharp tooth edges. Patients often arrive with poor oral hygiene and gum erosions. Gingivitis and oral infections are particularly common in persons infected with HIVirus. The dental providers can be cut and contaminate the patient through the abraded gums. Blood and saliva from the patient can likewise contaminate the provider through a hand wound. This is a two-way street for viral transmission. It happens with the hepatitis viruses A, B, and C. HIVirus will be no exception.

Ultrasonic dental drills produce mist particles of blood, tissue, and bone fragments. Not known is what risk this poses to persons with acne or other breaks in the skin. Health care workers contaminated by blood splashed on open lesions have developed AIDS, but these occurrences are rare. Do aerosolized particles pose a threat if deposited on dental instruments, supposedly sterilized, waiting for the next patient?

At one time oral surgeons represented one of the highest risk groups in America for acquiring the hepatitis B virus, upwards of 24%. Fortunately, hepatitis B vaccines have significantly reduced this risk. There is no such vaccine for HIV (which is much more lethal than hepatitis B). There will likely never be an AIDS vaccine.

Dentists should know the HIV status of their patients. Likewise, every health care provider should know the communicable status of each patient they may have exposure to. This view point is not shared by most critics of testing (most of whom do not find themselves at personal risk). Civil libertarians, who dare not sacrifice their own lives, will take exception to the inherent imperfections of this policy. The limits of discrimination should be set by the virus, not by lawyers.

Dental providers are now required to dress in cumbersome protective gear. Goggles and face shields are prone to fogging. Comfort and visibility are impaired. This contributes to inadvertent injuries. A negative HIV test (in some elective circumstances this test may need to be repeated) along with a careful medical and social history could allow for the use of less awkward gowning equipment and provide more proficient dentistry. The ease with which dental procedures are performed determines safety and results. HIV screening can be done efficiently and cost effectively using the same saliva discarded down the sink.

Dentists are understandably fearful and reluctant to perform elective procedures on known HIV-positive patients. This is true regardless of observing every available precaution. They are knowingly risking their lives (and the life of their spouse or partner). The procedure to the patient is rarely life-saving, but the potential risk to the provider is always life-threatening.

A patient has the right to know the HIV status of the dental provider; a patient has the right *not* to be placed at increased risk for AIDS. When a group of California dentists recently chose to disclose their HIV status they were publicly reprimanded and silenced by activists and their attorneys.

Most dental exposures to HIV are never recognized. I support the position, however unpopular, that it is exercising poor medical judgment for an HIV-negative dentist to treat an HIV-positive patient. Likewise, it is just as dangerous for an HIV-positive dentist to treat an HIV-negative patient. One can only wonder what it would be like for an HIV-positive dentist or hygienist to inform a patient that a fresh cut on the provider's hand had just leaked infected blood onto the abraded gums of the unaware patient. The shock and panic to the patient would be unimaginable. Saying nothing would be worse! Inherent in avoiding this calamity is an awareness of who is HIV-positive—the dental provider, the dental patient, you, me.

Most people who have been HIV tested and are positive go unreported. Many other people who are positive have never actually been tested. As of 1993 the prevalence rate of HIV in America was estimated to be 0.7% to 2.0%. Without performing public health this number cannot be verified. There is justification for The Federal Centers for Disease *Control* and *Prevention*, in conjunction with the American Dental Association, to set firm standardized policies to ensure public safety. Authorities must choose between putting the brakes on this epidemic (to save lives) or running for cover under the umbrella of political expediency. Why should saving lives be so unpopular? When mistakes are made let them be on the side of overcaution. AIDS has no cure. Fear and intimidation should never prevent what is medically sound and morally correct.

A dentist is someone prone to blood-borne disease. This person should know his or her HIV status, if for no other reason than to protect a spouse or sexual partner. This is common sense. This is love.

OPERAIDS

All truth passes through three steps.
First, it is ridiculed.
Second, it is violently opposed.
Third, it is accepted as being self-evident.

— *Arthur Schopenhauer*

23

What's with the space suit? Is my surgeon preparing to remove a gallbladder or be launched to the moon?

The surgeon is a physician who heals by the skilled use of the knife. In so doing there is a risk of co-mingling his or her blood with that of the patient. This risk is small but nonetheless more so than in any other field of medicine. In certain surgical sub-specialties the risk is particularly high, such as cardiovascular surgery and trauma surgery. Procedures that by their nature are confined to small spaces such as vaginal surgery, make injury more likely. Wherever there is exposure to sharp bony spikes, as might occur in orthopedic, thoracic, and oral surgery, there is greater risk for puncture wounds and skin tears. These injuries allow for transmission of blood-borne infections in either direction, from the patient to the doctor or from the doctor to the patient. It is reasonable to try to minimize any risk and if possible eliminate risk altogether. If you turn on an electric switch one thousand times and know that you may get electrocuted one chance out of a thousand, wouldn't you do everything in your power not to throw that switch, especially if you had already risked it nine hundred ninety-nine times?

Surgeons must be comfortable while operating. Good surgical results depend upon it. Our lives depend upon it. If surgical tools are not properly sterilized, if the operating amphitheater is not antiseptic, if your surgeon is weary—you may be in trouble. Hot, baggy gowns, occlusive masks, triple gloves, and fogging eye protection make for cumbersome and more difficult surgery.

Resurrected supposedly to protect health care providers from communicable diseases, *universal precautions* claim to be the perfect antiseptic antidiscriminator. Integrated into AIDS hospital policy these precautions now guarantee that all diseases are created equal. If practiced to the letter, these precautions might actually preclude the possibility of providing safer surgery for most patients. Adhering to these precautions protects hospitals from the crackdown of OSHA (Occupational Safety and Health Administration), and JCAHO (Joint Commission for the Accreditation of Healthcare Organizations). Robotically following these precautions also promotes a thriving rubber glove industry in Malaysia. What these universal precautions *fail* to do is to seriously challenge the AIDS epidemic. A review panel at the Johns Hopkins Medical Center, where universal precautions are stressed, found that 80% of needle-stick injuries are not preventable. Judiciously applied, universal precautions should *complement* rather than *substitute* for necessary HIV screening. Precautions without testing accomplish little, except to provide an infection control scapegoat for our unwillingness to accept the basic principles of epidemiology. The only effective means to prevent the spread of AIDS is to practice responsible infection control and epidemiology within the hospital and in the community outside of the hospital. We do neither!

Universal precautions remain the official party line for risk reduction in preventing the spread of HIV in the operating room. What are these universal precautions we entrust our lives to? The assumption made is that all bodily fluids are potentially infectious and therefore should be prevented from coming into contact with open wounds, skin rashes, and mucous membranes. Eye shields are worn to protect the eyes. Gloves are used to protect the skin of the hand. No one is to operate with any open sores or injuries of the skin. It is recommended wearing fluid-impervious gowns (even though these don't exist) and handling sharp instruments in such a way as to make injury impossible. These are certainly ideal goals. But are they realistic? To be truly protected one would have to wear a space suit impervious to any damage. Gloves are very delicate and easily tear. Needles and knives always have the advantage over rubber, latex, or vinyl. The longer the operation the more likely gloves will develop holes (up to 40% of the time in some studies). Most people have some kind of minor scratch, bruise, or injury somewhere on their body. Surgeons are no exception. If they were to stay out of the operating room each time they had some open wound on their body they would be performing very little surgery.

Routine is the mantra of the surgeon. Do it the same way every time and things become second nature, ensuring few errors. But how much do universal precautions interrupt the traditional way of doing things? At the very least these precautions slow things down. Speed is not the most important thing in the conduct of an operation, but the length of time a procedure takes is a significant risk factor. Prolonged anesthesia is associated with increased heart and lung complications. Prolonged surgery is associated with a significant increased risk of serious postoperative wound infections and pneumonia. The longer an operation takes the more opportunity there is for blood loss. These increased surgical complications are associated with an increased risk of death. **The AIDS epidemic complicates surgery for everyone.**

All patients now pay the price. Patients are frequently under anesthesia longer. A surgeon is compromised by a longer procedure. A surgeon's exhaustion may affect you or the case after you. As a complication of the HIV epidemic all surgical procedures are more difficult, more risky, and more costly. Most surgeons would prefer doing surgery the old way, the safer and faster way, if they could be supported by a negative HIV test and a careful medical and social history from the patient. A hip fracture, a heart attack, a deadly virus are all treated with the same precautions—not in accordance with the risk each one generates.

There are other possible risks in the operating room that universal precautions do not even address. Many procedures use high frequency oscillating equipment that creates an aerosol of blood and serum that sprays into the air. Some electrical and laser equipment produces a plume of smoke that has live virus particles still present. In some viral diseases this is already known to be a risk to the surgeon. For example, the human papilloma virus causes venereal warts. When these lesions are burned off an aerosol is produced. If inhaled the particulate can give rise to warts on the vocal cords and tracheobronchial tree of the surgeon, as well as everyone else in the operating suite. So far there have been no reports of this route of transmission of HIV, but blood-splash injuries causing HIV transmission to health care providers have been well documented. We are still in the learning curve of this disease and should not be surprised about the biologic behavior of this or any other micro-organism.

Universal precautions teach (preach) that all health care providers should wear gloves when examining each and every patient whenever there is a perceived risk of bodily fluid exposure. These precautions warn that every patient should be presumed HIV-positive and that there is always the potential for exposure. Now, one might wonder, how do we handle this circumstance when at any one time 98% of all HIV-positive people are not even hospitalized? Since when do the bodily secretions of an AIDS patient cease to be contagious when they leave the hospital? Does this mean we are all to wear gloves at restaurants and barber shops in case there is an unexpected mishap? The vast majority of HIV-infected people are without symptoms and not hospitalized. Under these circumstances universal precautions are completely ignored. Universal precautions observed in the hospital warn us of a lurking danger but do little to affect the epidemic.

The availability of HIV screening in 1985 allowed for much safer transfusion of blood products. As a consequence, for each case of AIDS now acquired in a hospital setting there are over 500 cases acquired outside of hospitals. The real precautions that should be taken are universal HIV testing and reporting. This should be applied both in the hospital and in the community. A careful medical history in conjunction with HIV screening are the most important safety measures to practice. This is called common sense and it's time has come.

The general surgeon is injured on the job six to eight times a year. The professional life of a surgeon is forty years (approximately 300 injuries). If the prevalence of AIDS in a community is 1%, three of the injuries have the potential for transmitting the HIVirus. Thus there is about one in one hundred chances of that surgeon potentially acquiring the infection in his or her lifetime through a surgical injury. If the surgeon practices in an area where the prevalence of HIV positivity is 10% the risk would be one in ten. Some inner-city emergency rooms already have a higher prevalence than that. Soon this may be the norm throughout the country, just as it already is in much of Africa. **The risk of HIV to a surgeon is not minor despite all the universal precautions one can muster.**

Cardiovascular surgeons, with whom I have personally discussed the matter of intraoperative injuries, tell me that at least one puncture wound or laceration occurs in every 30 surgical cases. Some have indicated that the incidence is as high as one in every ten cases. This same group of doctors is affected by a high hepatitis B exposure rate. It would be fair to assume that they share a similarly high risk for HIV exposure and that this risk will increase with time as more of the population becomes infected. Once again, because testing is not mandatory, the actual risk is unknown. Fortunately a vaccine is now available to prevent hepatitis B. No such vaccine is expected for HIV.

As medical students we were taught the importance of a thorough history and physical examination and appropriate laboratory studies. The benefit of this is improved patient care. Every physician should be aware if a patient has other underlying diseases that could complicate surgery or compromise medical treatment. The politics of AIDS has changed this time-honored concept of medical education and health care. **The most dangerous infection of my lifetime is still struggling to be recognized as an infectious disease.**

Testing would identify patients who are HIV-positive and who might expect postoperative complications as a consequence of their immune suppression. A positive HIV test in some circumstances might influence whether an operative procedure should even be performed. Someone with advanced HIV disease but without AIDS-related symptoms might want to avoid certain procedures such as heart surgery, organ transplant, or joint replacement. The patient and health care provider could make a more informed decision regarding surgery.

Testing also identifies risk to the health care provider. The mere mention of this fact inflames some AIDS activists who are unwilling to accept the reality that a positive HIV test has medical significance to the health care provider. In the bigger picture of how this epidemic is being fueled the significance seems small. Nonetheless, to the individual health care provider, the danger is real. Many health care providers have already lost their lives as a consequence of treating patients who are HIV-positive. The patients they treated had no chance to survive. The provider who becomes infected will have no effective treatment either. If the provider should become inadvertently infected and is not aware, he/she may transmit this virus to a spouse, lover, or unborn child.

If a nurse should accidentally be stabbed with a blood-contaminated needle, under most circumstances it is necessary to obtain _permission_ from the patient to obtain an HIV test. Imagine when permission is denied. Imagine what it is like living with the fear of possibly being infected as a result of this needle-stick exposure and possibly infecting your spouse through sex or shared secretions. For the next three to six months this nurse's life is turned upside down because the patient to whom he or she was providing care refused permission to be HIV tested—a test that would not change that patient's HIV status. Now imagine this nurse is married to a civil libertarian, a proponent of this patient's right "not to be tested." Imagine how different this situation suddenly appears. Imagine how short-sighted we have all become!

Activists who decry pre-operative testing for HIV bring up several arguments to support their position for not testing (a position I believe compromises the lives of health care providers). They argue, "We live in a sea of infectious agents, therefore universal precautions are the only logical protection." While it is true that there is a multitude of infectious organisms, we are certain that the HIVirus is a particularly vicious killer for which there is unequivocally no cure. The mortality approaches 100%. The other common transmittable agents are of lesser virulence. There are measures to control, treat, or eradicate them.

Another argument frequently used against HIV screening is that the knowledge of the HIV status does not change the behavior of the surgeon. Reality is that most surgeons I have spoken with do change their behavior significantly. Above all they slow down considerably to avoid injuries. Universal precautions that are usually practiced with a cavalier attitude are suddenly adhered to religiously. In the best of all worlds one might expect that this would be done in all cases anyway. We don't live in the best of all worlds. Let's not make it the worst of all worlds. Human nature being what it is takes short cuts, takes the easier, more comfortable, more accustomed path when we are not directly confronted with visible danger. Operating in double gowns under hot operating lights gets pretty uncomfortable. A shield to protect the eyes, especially in a person who already wears glasses, fogs up. You cannot see—a real handicap for a surgeon! Passing instruments from nurse to surgeon is so traditionally ritualistic that not to pass one class of instruments (sharps) versus another becomes confusing and troublesome. Following all the universal precaution guidelines prolongs and complicates each and every operation. Patients remain under anesthesia longer. A surgeon is compromised by a longer procedure. A surgeon's exhaustion may affect you or the case after you.

The next argument advanced is that it takes several months

for the HIV test to become positive after the initial exposure. A negative test does not necessarily mean that you have a patient who is free of the virus. There is a "window period" when a person may be highly contagious but not yet test positive. In any biologic situation there is a bell curve. We live with a certain degree of uncertainty. Life has its risks. The risk of HIV exposure can be minimized but never entirely eliminated. Most HIV-positive individuals would be identified if all were tested.

AIDS is lethal. AIDS talk is hardball. Now that some civil libertarians are sufficiently heated up, a final point deserves mention. Elective (not emergency) surgery provided to HIV-positive patients should preferably be performed only by HIV-positive surgeons. The number of HIV-positive surgeons and the number of HIV-positive patients will escalate as the epidemic progresses. As the virus spreads unchecked in the population more health care providers will become infected as a consequence of their occupation as well as their private life exposures. A surgeon is more likely to be HIV infected today than at any time in the past. The exact numbers are not known because we are not doing the appropriate screening. There is absolutely no reason to risk unnecessarily the life of a surgeon or anyone else. **Any opportunity to avoid a single infection should not be lost.**

Under most circumstances an HIV-positive surgeon should not operate on an HIV-negative patient. This is especially true without the patient's informed consent. Mathematical models have suggested the risk to patients in this setting to be very low. However, because there is no universal surveillance and because symptoms may take many years to develop, the actual risk is not known. Anything above zero is too high!

Hepatitis B and C viruses are the closest blood-borne infectious models to HIVirus. The risk of transmitting any of these three viruses from an infected health care worker to a susceptible individual depends upon a number of factors including the type of procedure, the infection control precautions observed, and the individual skill and technique of the health care provider. *Even more significant is the infectious status of the provider.* A resident surgeon at a University of California affiliated hospital infected 19 of his patients with hepatitis B virus during surgical procedures. 13% of the patients he operated on became infected. The surgeon did not violate standard infection control procedures. Similarly, a cardiac surgeon in Spain, known to have chronic hepatitis C, infected five of his patients during surgery. All five of these patients underwent heart valve replacements. It is believed the injuries occurred while closing the sternum with wires. The surgeon estimated an incidence of 20 skin injuries to himself per 100 procedures. Tying the chest wall with wires is associated with a high rate of glove perforation. This invariably leads to contact of the surgeon's blood with the patient's open wound. Had these surgeons been HIV-positive, all 24 patients could have been silently infected with the AIDS virus.

Every person, including every surgeon, should know his or her HIV status, if for no other reason than to protect his or her spouse or sexual partner where the risk of transmission may be many fold greater than in the operating room. One study projected a significant cost of testing all surgeons. The study was based on comparing the number of AIDS cases that would be prevented to the cost of testing. It projected a high cost for testing thousands of surgeons in order to prevent just a few cases of AIDS. It ignored the fact that each case of AIDS becomes an index case for the next case and the next case. It ignored the fact that mass screening could be done at a fraction of the cost of individual testing. Saliva testing could be done even less expensively. How many more lives must be lost? **How much more suffering does it take to make the practice of public health cost effective?**

Surgery is inherently risky. Now add to the equation prolonged surgery and anesthesia as a consequence of universal precautions. Now add to the equation an HIV-infected surgeon or scrub nurse. Who said things would get better?

CALL IT WHAT YOU WANT !!

24

*I do not mind what language an opera is sung in
so long as it is a language I don't understand.*
— *Sir Edward Appleton*

A positive HIV test should stand alone as an AIDS defining diagnosis. Anything less is voodoo medicine.

A deadly pandemic was unfolding by the early 1980's. No infectious agent was yet implicated. A few San Francisco doctors termed the new enigmatic disease BANDAID (Bay Area Newly Described Acquired Immune Disorder). Others coined the new illness GRIDS (Gay Related Immune Deficiency Syndrome). AIDS is now the widely accepted acronym (Acquired Immune Deficiency Syndrome). In Spanish and French it is known as SIDA.

ARC (AIDS Related Complex) is a term frequently used to describe early symptoms of this ailment. This includes low grade fevers, weight loss, and swollen lymph nodes. All ARC patients eventually become more symptomatic and die of AIDS. ARC patients are contagious. ARC patients have AIDS. They are in the intermediate phase of illness and in the late stage of life. ARC is the medical synonym for Denial. ARC allays fears, especially that of the patient. The temporary calm is marred with a false sense

of hope and a frustrating wait for the inevitable. Hope slips to disappointment. ARC slips to AIDS. Public health services lapse into coma and the patient slips into the grave.

The term ARC has no clinical value and should be discarded to the Archives of Medical Confusion. ARC is AIDS. Breast cancer is breast cancer, even if the malignancy has not yet metastasized to the liver or brain. No other medical condition is subjected to the same institutional denial as AIDS.

In January of 1993 the Federal Centers for Disease Control redefined AIDS from its previous 1987 classification. The initial definition included a positive HIV test or a syndrome of weight loss, fevers, and swollen lymph nodes (prior to the availability of HIV testing) accompanied by any or several of the following:

- Opportunistic infection such as pneumocystis carinii pneumonia, cryptococcal meningitis, disseminated coccidioidiomycosis and histoplasmosis, toxoplasmosis, nocardiosis, extraintestinal strongyloidosis, etc.
- Kaposi's sarcoma (KS)
- AIDS related malignancies, particularly lymphomas
- HIV-related neuropathy
- Progressive multifocal leukoencephalopathy (PML)
- Severe wasting (30% of muscle mass)
- CMV retinitis
- Disseminated tuberculosis
- Disseminated atypical mycobacteria (avium or kansasii)
- Widespread herpes simplex
- Salmonella septicemia, recurrent
- Invasive candidiasis of esophagus, trachea, bronchi, or lungs

The revised January 1993 criteria included the following additions:

- Absolute CD4 count < 200
- Helper/suppressor ratio (CD4/CD8) < 0.14
- Invasive cervical carcinoma
- Recurrent (2 or more episodes) pneumonia
- Pulmonary tuberculosis

A CD4 count is the laboratory measurement of the number of helper T-lymphocytes in the peripheral blood. This is also commonly referred to as the T4 count. These cells represent the arm of the immune system that is initially attacked by the human immuno-deficiency retrovirus. The count is used as a clinical guide to the extent of disease. It is relied upon to determine when to initiate antiretroviral therapy and when to consider prophylaxis against opportunistic infections. A lower CD4 count generally indicates more advanced disease.

As noted above, guidelines from the CDC were revised to include a CD4 count of less than 200 as an AIDS defining diagnosis. The normal CD4 count in most laboratories is at least 600 and often much greater. Hypothetically, patient #1, who is HIV-positive and asymptomatic with a CD4 Count of 180, would be defined as having AIDS. Patient #2, who is also HIV-positive and also without symptoms and having a CD4 count of 220, would not meet the CDC criteria for AIDS. There is enough variability in CD4 testing that simply repeating the tests at different laboratories could reverse which of these two patients would be officially defined as having AIDS. This is nonsense. The cold fact is that both patients are far advanced in their illness. Both patients are contagious and both patients deserve to know the truth about their illness and prognosis. They do not benefit from institutional denial. They need the support of family, friends, and health care agencies. Both patients have AIDS!

Patients denying that they have terminal disease is not unusual. However, when health care providers and agencies promote this denial and refuse to acknowledge a deadly disease, no one benefits. Institutional denial will neither save lives nor slow the epidemic. Watching a disease devour a patient and refusing to recognize its existence has no medical justification. When the CDC finally adjusted its criteria for AIDS defining illness in 1993, to include a CD4 count of less than 200, the AIDS incidence doubled overnight. This was a large step for statistics but an even larger step for truth.

WE HAVE BASEBALL FOR THAT

25

Mark Twain once commented, "The greatest lie is a statistical lie."

Health authorities are locked into tabulating statistics of late stage disease. Instead, they should be responsible for preventing transmission in early stage disease. Counting the dead won't bring them back. Let's start counting the living!

Perhaps there is good reason why life comes before liberty and the pursuit of happiness. AIDS patients know that there is no happiness in taking nine different toxic medications daily, enduring repeated injections, always feeling short of breath, living with constant diarrhea, and being too weak to feed or dress themselves. All the while, they know they won't get well. This is what we need to prevent!

HIVirus does not discriminate. It does not care if you are man or woman, a few days old or one hundred years old. You can be an unborn fetus infected in utero. Your lover is not immune and neither are you. Each new case becomes the index case for another human-to-human transmission. Each new case will result in death.

AIDS claims one new victim in the world every

7 to 10 seconds. Included are our children, siblings, parents, friends and neighbors. Each of them was infected by a virus that once found refuge in someone else. This is a person-to-person disease. With the exception of the air we breathe, nothing has quite connected us like AIDS. We don't think about each breath. We don't think about each lost person. The AIDS quilt is pieced with newly sewn patches in remembrance of loved ones. It will soon cover the face of the earth, as each name becomes more and more faceless.

The primary goal of public health services, to preserve and protect the health of the citizenry, has been trampled upon in this epidemic. The basic principles of epidemiology that apply to all contagious diseases have been cast aside when applied to AIDS. HIV surveillance ranges from totally inadequate to totally absent. The adequacy of surveillance defines the adequacy of intervention—both are a dismal (and deadly) failure. Political rhetoric and legal intimidation have replaced sound medical judgment. Concerned about preserving certain ill-defined civil liberties, we are neglectful of preserving human lives. Where is the value in gay rights without a healthy gay population? **How much do any rights matter to a dead person or to a society that is terminally ill?**

In his remarkable epilogue, *And The Band Played On,* Randy Shilts correctly warned against politicizing this contagion. Is the band now dead as well? So fearful of stepping into a political minefield, health providers have willfully permitted a medical disaster to go unabated. Controlling the transmission of this disease is the only available option we presently have at controlling this epidemic. This certainly includes AIDS education, but not at the exclusion of stringent public health policies. We need a workable guidance system that coordinates education with surveillance and intervention.

NASA could not have hoped to land a man on the moon just by firing rocket boosters aimlessly toward the heavens. Controlling the global AIDS epidemic is a feat far more difficult than a moon-landing. This requires individuals with authority who will not be deterred by confusing statutes and empty recommendations. Common sense law and humanitarian goals must supersede any individual's privacy rights. Expect unpleasant choices. Individual rights can conflict with the welfare and safety of others, as does the right to recklessly drive a speeding car through a busy intersection.

It is a futile effort to try stopping the spread of any communicable disease, and especially one so insidious, if it is not known who is infected. Since there is no panacea, we can afford no mistakes. Our present "no look, no ask, no do" policy on AIDS has never been applied to any other contagious disease. Our failure to contain this epidemic should be no surprise. The need for change is clubbing us over the head. Let's pray it jars loose our common sense.

HIV is a silent bullet, often leaving no clues as to who fired or when. Universal screening or testing or surveillance (take your pick) is an absolute necessity for containment. It should have been instituted years ago. To be effective, testing cannot be done anonymously. All positive cases must be reported and followed-up by health authorities. Testing should not be done solely for statistical purposes—we have baseball for that.

To challenge reporting laws in Colorado, hundreds of infected individuals submitted the name "Nancy Reagan" on their test reports. Many of those who protested still displayed ambivalence by leaving their correct address, recognizing the responsibility of partner notification. Many of these "Nancy Reagan" cases and their unreported contacts have since died of AIDS. They protected the virus, not themselves.

One role of government is to *enact* laws to protect public welfare. As a twist of fate would have it, we now need government to *prevent* laws and regulations that shackle public health authorities from performing their proper functions. AIDS prevention is in everyone's interest. The right to quality life, with all the medical and social assistance this entails, must be guaranteed for those who are infected. But more importantly, the right of the uninfected to remain uninfected is paramount.

Treatable diseases such as gonorrhea, syphilis, and tuberculosis are reportable to local public health departments. These departments are then responsible for notifying contacts of infected individuals and assisting in therapy. This breaks the chain of communicability. These diseases are rarely lethal. An incredible irony is that HIV is lethal, contagious, and only sporadically reported.

As of 1992 only 24 states required reporting of all positive HIV tests by name, but with no mandate that partners be notified. Ten additional states required reporting be done anonymously, guaranteeing no partner notification by health authorities. A North Carolina study pointed out that when partner notification is left to the infected individual only 6% reported notifying their partner(s). Remember, these are the partners of a deadly, incurable disease. Estimates are that over 50% of the women in this country who are HIV-infected do not know their risk.

Instead of quietly observing on the sidelines, feminist groups must demand action from public health services. It is time for all women to wake up, stand up, and be counted. Over half of the babies born with HIV in America have mothers who are unaware of their own status. These HIV-infected babies will all die. They will also become orphans (if they outlive their mothers). *Failed public health policy is not just about AIDS, it is also about child neglect and endangerment!*

As evidenced by blind surveillance studies, the emphasis is *not* to know who is infected. By not informing those individuals who test positive, our entrusted health authorities are giving up on any chance of prevention. Blinded AIDS surveillance fails to promote the traditional public health objectives of early treatment and disruption of transmission. It is unconscionable to think that anyone would do blinded screening studies in high risk communities, particularly at inner-city venereal disease and prenatal clinics, and not inform those who are infected. If there is any conspiracy that has ever been associated with AIDS, it would be to allow many of the poor, frequently Black and Hispanic inner-city victims to go unidentified and untreated. This is the green light permitting further spread of AIDS in these communities. 80% of the heterosexual spread of AIDS through 1994 was in minority communities, far in excess of their percentage of the general population. Greater then 70% of the HIV-infected women in this country are Black or Hispanic. These are the women taking the biggest punch at the hands of public health neglect. Many are unaware they are infected (and dying). Would someone at least call 9-1-1!

In New York City, mothers of HIV-infected newborns were often not informed of test results. The argument for this being that mothers had the legal right to not know the status of their child or themselves. This is *legal insanity!* The failure to notify and counsel seropositives and offer treatment to babies and their mothers fails every test of morality. Testing and failing to notify treats human subjects like laboratory animals. The 1948 Declaration of Geneva as well as the Declaration of Helsinki emphasized that the interest and well being of the patient is paramount to any scientific research. The policy of blinded HIV surveillance makes the sickening Tuskegee experiment with untreated syphilis, which lasted until 1972, look civil in comparison.

AIDS reporting most often occurs at the latest stages of disease, years after infection. Because we are capable of screening and conscientiously choose not to do so, most of the time period of communicability of AIDS is intentionally and outright ignored. Prevention is prevented by default—by doing nothing.

The CDC publishes guidelines periodically redefining AIDS. These guidelines are followed in all 50 states and by all county health departments. They are often referenced in other parts of the world. As a consequence of CDC classification, the actual incidence of AIDS is arbitrary, and more subject to committee changes than to reality. By using incorrect criteria to define AIDS, this government agency is knowingly sanctioning a late diagnosis. This inevitably leads to late or no intervention. I do not believe this is done by conspiracy or malice. I do, however, believe it has been a policy based on political expediency that falsely lowered the AIDS incidence (and still does). **To ignore the first 8 to 10 years of this disease and its contagious implications defies all logic.** The CDC may more appropriately be the acronym for *Conscientiously Denying Care* (my wife just informed me I'll never get a job there!). Fortunately, these arbitrary guidelines have recently been amended in the direction of more appropriate early diagnosis. But why not go all the way with the truth? What are we protecting, and from whom? The public and infected individuals should know the truth about this disease and what to expect.

HIV infection at any stage is what is relevant, whether or not it is labeled AIDS. HIV-positive means HIV contagious and it means AIDS. Asymptomatic gonorrhea is still gonorrhea. A small and silent cancerous lesion of the lung is still lung cancer. I know of no other medical circumstance where there has been such denial by the health care community, and no illness where there has been such consistent suffering and hopelessness.

HIV-infected people don't benefit from institutionalized denial; they need medical help and community support. Likewise, society requires the full cooperation of all HIV-positive individuals to combat this pandemic. Identification of each index case and all secondary and tertiary cases is mandatory to disrupt the chain of transmission. Everyone infected, regardless of classification by CDC criteria, must be identified and counseled for the remainder of their lives. This is Basic Epidemiology 101.

I do not believe the AIDS epidemic is shrouded by any government or scientific conspiracy. As a physician who treats AIDS patients, no one has ever approached me to cooperate with any such intrigue. Everyone wants a cure. However, an extraterrestrial, not familiar with modern behavior of the human species and observing this epidemic going unchallenged, might make an erroneous conclusion that there must be a conspiracy of sorts. How could the human species suddenly allow itself to be killed off so easily? Have reason and common sense been sapped from their spirit?

The unwillingness to follow normal public health procedures is a medical blunder of astronomical proportions. I believe this mistake has its roots in progressively adversarial societies where self-preservation and individual rights are perceived as separate from the common good. We behave by protecting our individual selves first and our species last. Invariably, in group discussions about AIDS, questions are focused on how an individual can protect oneself from infection, rarely on how communities can be protected. Not unlike violent crime, what happens across the city is someone else's problem. Soon we will be that victim across the city, or the next HIV-converter.

PLANES, TRAINS, AND TUBERCULAIDS

26

*My humanity is bound up in yours,
so we can only be human together.*

— *Archbishop Desmond Tutu*
(Nobel Peace Prize, 1984)

It suffocated Chopin. They called it consumption. Eleanor Roosevelt carried it to her grave. Tuberculosis was not recognized until after her death.

An airline stewardess contracted tuberculosis. Her risk factor (your risk factor) was an infected passenger. Her flights depart New York City.

In the 1970's medical students were taught that tuberculosis would be eradicated from the United States towards the end of the 20th century. This great achievement would be attributed to improved treatment protocols and to aggressive case finding through public health intervention. We are now nearing the end of the 20th century and TB elimination has *not* occurred. Ooops!

By 1984 he steady decline of TB actually began to reverse. It has been on the rise ever since. This reversal has very much to do with the coexistent AIDS epidemic. The socioeconomic problems plaguing this country are not helping. I believe the general health of a nation can be judged by its ability to control tuberculosis. **Our country's health is failing.**

People with AIDS are fueling the transmission of tuberculosis into the general population. Many nations attribute a resurgence of tuberculous pneumonia to the direct failure of controlling AIDS. An awareness of who is HIV-positive would warn of this complicating problem of TB. HIV-awareness would permit earlier identification and treatment of tuberculosis and curtail the spread of this mycobacterial infection that is killing both HIV-infected and HIV-noninfected people.

"All aboard . . . Next stop, your doctor's office." On January 23, 1996, by national announcement, Amtrak alerted train passengers from two Eastern seaboard routes to consult their physicians. It came to Amtrak's attention that a passenger had been ill with active cavitary tuberculosis. Other train passengers may have been exposed. But can we really expect Amtrak to know the health status of its passengers? Are subway authorities in Chicago, Paris, or London responsible for keeping medical records and screening all passengers for tuberculosis or other communicable diseases? What about grocery stores, banks, or indoor sporting arenas? 99.99% of random exposures to tuberculosis go unnoticed until the person exposed becomes ill, the source remaining a mystery.

"Please bring your seat to a full upright position and fasten your safety belt." Exposure to tuberculosis on airplanes is difficult to document since symptoms do not develop immediately and passengers disperse upon landing. Nonetheless, this source of transmission has already been recognized for passengers and crew members. Limited ventilation in closed compartments for prolonged periods of time intensify the risk of transmitting air-borne pathogens, TB included. One can expect that the risk of airline travel exposure, although low, will steadily climb as the TB epidemic spreads unchecked. It is *not* the role of United or Delta Airlines to screen passengers for TB. Controlling tuberculosis in the general population is the recognized responsibility of public health officials. They are entrusted to intervene whenever the public's health is jeopardized. They must now act on that responsibility. Controlling tuberculosis requires controlling

AIDS. Controlling AIDS requires public health officials knowing who is HIV-positive.

Persons infected with HIV are ten to thirty times more likely to develop tuberculosis. AIDS patients respond poorly when newly exposed to tuberculosis. As a consequence of their immuno-suppressed condition, they also have a greater than 100-fold chance of reactivating an old or dormant tuberculosis infection. TB is the principal killer of HIV-positive people in developing countries.

HIV and TB have spilled into the homeless and helpless populations of the world, making both contagions more difficult to control. Nearly half the world's refugees have already been infected with tuberculosis. In the United States it is more difficult to alleviate the homeless problem and reestablish persons back into main stream society when they are severely debilitated from either or both of these deadly diseases. Containing the AIDS and tuberculosis epidemics would give humankind greater opportunity to address other social ailments, of which there are plenty.

The control of tuberculosis now requires universal screening for HIV and a *living and breathing* public health system. Common sense dictates that better control of the AIDS epidemic would also better control the tuberculosis epidemic. Controlling the tuberculosis epidemic will also allow persons infected with HIV to live longer—one less opportunistic infection to worry about!

According to Hiroshi Nakajima, MD, Director General of the World Health Organization, "Not only has TB returned, it has upstaged its own horrible legacy." With the death rate from tuberculosis sharply rising, WHO was prompted in 1993 to declare TB a global health emergency. In 1995 TB claimed 3 million lives—more than in any other year of recorded history. WHO now projects 90 million new cases during the present decade and a staggering 500 million cases over the next 50 years. Has this watchdog organization given up all hope of containing tuberculosis (and AIDS)?

The 1990's was supposed to be the decade that would close the chapter on tuberculosis. A mismanaged AIDS epidemic has prevented this closure. An awareness of who is

HIV-positive would enable health care providers to warn and screen patients for the increased risk of developing TB. Rapid treatment of TB prevents the spread of this pathogen and saves lives. HIV is out of control. TB is out of control. **The world's health is failing.**

In recent years the tuberculosis bacilli (mycobacteria hominis) has become more resistant to the same conventional treatment protocols that were once supposed to eradicate this organism. The death toll from multi-drug resistant TB has now included a number of health care providers. It is estimated that 90% of cases of drug resistant TB will occur in those infected with HIV. In New York City, where AIDS is particularly rampant, it is estimated that one in every six people has already been infected with tuberculosis. Many of these cases are actively infected, not on treatment, and highly contagious. Many also have multi-drug resistant strains. The multi-drug resistant TB patients are rarely cured, remain contagious, and require strict and often life-long isolation. Because these strains of tuberculosis are highly resistant to conventional safer therapy, the required substitute drug regimens are often associated with many more toxic side effects. The cost of caring for a single patient with resistant TB has been estimated at over $200,000 per year.

Treatment failure is the rule when treating resistant TB strains. The mortality rate from resistant TB ranges from 80% to 90%. Fearful for their own health and of spreading resistant tuberculosis to their families, health care providers are very reluctant to care for these people. It is rumored that in New York City even antidiscrimination lawyers have declined to make personal visits! Many of those infected with resistant tuberculosis live on the streets or in subway stations or in crowded shelters. Homeless people are often very ill. They need our help to get well. We need their help to control both the AIDS and tuberculosis epidemics.

Unlike AIDS, TB is transmitted through relatively casual contact by aerosolized droplets. Even though HIV has been shown to be harbored in the lungs, mostly in cells known as pulmonary macrophages, there is yet to be any proof that

HIV can be transmitted via respiratory particles. This includes patients who may be dual-infected with HIV and TB (or with other respiratory infections that AIDS patients might acquire such as pneumocystis carinii, atypical mycobacteria, and fungi).

Pray the HIVirus never spreads like the common cold or flu! If there was ever a welcome blessing with this disease, it would be here. HIV is a lentivirus. Other viruses of this class that affect animals, such as sheep and goats, are spread horizontally by biting and sharing saliva. There is also concern of possible air-borne route of lentivirus transmission in animals, but this has not yet been proven. Should this respiratory mode of transmission ever occur with HIVirus as a consequence of viral mutation, the AIDS epidemic would explode to include everyone within several decades. Humankind would be teetering that much closer to the brink of extinction.

A FOOL AND HIS MONEY

We have first raised the dust,
and then complain we cannot see.
— *George Berkeley*

27

A cheeseburger costs 89 cents. Add a bag of fries and a medium-sized drink and you're up to $2.49.

A postage stamp is 32 cents. To express mail a parcel would cost more than an AIDS test. The saliva used to moisten the stamps can be HIV tested for less than $2.00.

A long distance phone call can be several dollars. The cost of calling a friend is the cost of protecting a friend.

Movie tickets for two cost about $15.00. This is more than the cost of performing 3 blood or 7 saliva AIDS tests.

A nice dinner for two could screen 15 saliva specimens for HIVirus. Include wine and it's 25 saliva tests. Include a tip and 35 persons could be tested (I'm a big tipper).

The four year cost of one student's tuition at Stanford University could pay for the testing of the school's entire student body. If that student goes on to medical school the entire populations of Juneau, Fairbanks, and Anchorage, Alaska, could be tested.

The cost of the O.J. Simpson Trial could purchase over 5,500,000 saliva tests. This is larger than the combined populations of Wyoming, Montana, Idaho, the Dakotas, New Mexico, and Nevada.

One Trident submarine (the US has at least five) costs the American tax payer over 3 billion dollars to build and maintain. This could test all of North and South America.

The repair bill caused by Hurricane Andrew could test the population of the entire world (twice).

AIDS monetarists will take exception. These are the people who count the money but don't treat the patients. Their business is not to measure suffering. They have no vision of an epidemic that is not colored green.

I must inform the reader that this has been the most difficult chapter for me to write. It requires placing a price tag on your life, on my life, and on the happiness of our children.

No economist will be able to measure the social crisis that is impending. No economist will be able to calculate the economic devastation that is impending. No economist can count that high. The cost of continuing to look the other way will be catastrophic.

The yearly per capita federal expense for AIDS prevention is $2.95. The estimated annual cost to treat a person with late-stage AIDS is $75,000. For some patients it is much greater due to incredibly expensive medications and prolonged hospital care. A Milwaukee hospital-based study concludes that the mean lifetime cost of caring for children with HIV is $418,863. None of these children survive! AIDS is a preventable, communicable disease. None of these children (or their mothers) should have been infected.

Half of nonsurgical beds in some inner-city hospitals are already occupied by AIDS patients. People with HIV infections now occupy 4-7% of all hospital beds in the USA—not a single person with AIDS has ever been cured. Most are no longer working and will never return to work. It is already estimated that the indirect cost from lost productivity and wages from AIDS-related illness is 7 times greater than direct medical costs. Canada is also experiencing the premature loss of many of its young people at their productive peaks. The staggering economic impact of AIDS is increasing relative to all other diseases throughout the world. In the African nation of Uganda the AIDS epidemic is so rampant that some companies hire and train two workers for every position, with the hope that one worker will remain healthy.

AZT and other antiretrovirals used in combination can cost upwards of $1,200 per month. Drugs to prevent fungal infections can cost up to $18 per pill per day. Once treatment of any established opportunistic infection begins the costs really skyrocket. Patients with CMV retinitis often require daily and lifelong intravenous therapy, costing thousands of dollars a week, even as an outpatient. Intravenous hyperalimentation (for those too weak to feed themselves) also costs thousands of dollars per week. **None will live long enough to see the final bill.**

Newer drugs, whether or not they demonstrate benefit, will translate into even more expensive therapy. Labs and x-rays and scans are already very expensive. It is estimated that the newer tests that measure viral load (concentration of virus in blood) will cost at least $150-$300 per test. Once hospitalized, all bets are off on costs.

AIDS care is paid for by private insurance and federal, state, and county funds, i.e. tax dollars. Those few fortunate enough to have a large nest egg could see it crack. No amount of money can save anyone. As the AIDS epidemic expands, private insurance rates will continue to escalate and all government funds will be depleted. Budgets remaining for everything else will be inadequate. Financial resources in Washington are already depleted, and not even because of AIDS.

Are we prepared to fund the most expensive medical crisis of all time? Federal grants for researching most diseases are becoming scarce. This once rich nation has many streets filled with gangs and drug addicts. The homeless shelters are crowded and the food lines are long. Public health facilities face closure. Roads and bridges, the infrastructure of this nation, are in their worst shape since the industrial revolution. The social fabric of America is torn. Homelessness, racial tension, and massive loss of good jobs are tearing society to shreds. Even physicians are losing their jobs! The spirit of

America is evaporating.

Now here come the medical economists, explaining how AIDS testing (and AIDS prevention) is too costly. They tell us that resources are better spent on treating an incurable disease, rather than on preventing that disease from ever occurring. **They tell us we cannot afford to stay alive.**

Statistical studies are empty of compassion and blind to the future. They are often selectively designed to prove cost inefficiency. Cost analysis by many of these AIDS statisticians completely ignores the reality that AIDS is an epidemic. Each case identified today is multiplied into many cases tomorrow. The numbers are not static. Every link in the chain of transmission must be broken. Yet, we are advised to roll over and do nothing, not to identify those infected—it would cost too much. Some studies that attempt to disprove the cost/benefit of testing are actually funded by tax dollars, the same dollars that could be appropriately spent providing public health services.

There are studies pointing out (incorrectly) the cost inefficiency of screening many groups, including health care workers. One such published study attempts to prove that testing all surgeons in the USA would result in expenditures of $458,000,000 per year of life saved. This number is based on wildly exaggerated estimates of testing costs, unnecessary pretest counseling for mass screening, unfounded knowledge of how many surgeons are infected, and what the true risk of exposure to patients is. Incidentally, a hospital I am affiliated with would perform the test for its employees and medical staff for free! Hospitals already screen for hepatitis B and tuberculosis at no cost to the health care worker. In the study's analysis 141,646 surgeons would require testing. Our government can test military recruits at $4.00 per test. Testing of these surgeons should cost less than $600,000. This minor expenditure would identify HIV-positive surgeons and allow them early medical intervention. Their patients and sexual partners could also be afforded protection. This same study pointed out that an unidentified, infected surgeon would have a 0.9% chance of infecting a sexual partner. The true incidence would be much greater. Even so, I wonder if the authors of this study would accept a 0.9% risk of transmitting a lethal, incurable disease to one of their own loved ones?

A thousand tests might identify only 7 infected surgeons today. Even identifying one would be reason enough to test. Three years from now it might be 20 or 30 infected surgeons per thousand tests (who knows?). The incorrect dollar amount often used in calculating the cost of performing an HIV blood test is $50.00 per test. The true cost is closer to $4.00 per test. Is $4,000 or $50,000 or $100,000 worth spending to identify seven infected surgeons? Yes, yes, and yes! The argument used for not testing is that most of these surgeons who are infected are unlikely to infect their patients anyway. Do we ignore those few that will get infected? Do we allow those few to carry the HIV torch to others? Soon the few become many. That's how this epidemic works. Even more importantly, surgeons are people with lives outside the hospital. Not only can they infect patients, but they can infect their spouse, sexual partner, or newborn child.

What about the cost of $50.00 per test? Mass blood screening by the military is done at $4.00 per test. This cuts the cost over 90%. Mass screening by private or government-funded labs could do the same. My own investigating, calling hospital and private labs, revealed per test cost to be $28.00, $14.00, $20.00, and, $13.67. I was also informed that contracted insurance companies paid considerably less. Every lab indicated that the reagent costs needed to do the testing could be less if more simultaneous testing was done. More recently saliva testing and even urine testing have been developed. With these more simple tests done in mass, the costs could be further reduced when performed by nonprofit public health agencies. The sensitivity of saliva and urine screening approaches that of blood testing. These tests have received wider use in other countries.

Assume 300 million Americans are blood tested at $4.00 per test. This would amount to 1.2 billion dollars. The daily interest on the national debt is $800 million. 36 hours worth of interest on the national debt could HIV test this entire nation. There are many Americans looking for work. I can't imagine a better way for the federal government to put people back to work then by funding a program of AIDS prevention. The money spent on testing would provide jobs for people and enhance the security of this nation. Saliva and urine testing might be considered in follow-up screening programs. Epidemiologists are trained to plan and implement such programs. These experts are getting rusty!

This nation still does not have a legal requirement or even a firm recommendation for premarital HIV testing. The economic rationale is that it might be too expensive to protect a spouse or newborn. The experts again point out how many thousands of dollars would be spent to identify a single infection. They fail to mention how each of these infections, going unnoticed, will spread. **They fail to mention the billions of dollars spent on therapy that doesn't work!**

Tracing contacts is critical to containing this epidemic. Presently we don't even know who most of the index cases are. We don't routinely test and we seldomly report cases unless diagnosed as full-blown AIDS. Contact notification is weighted down in legal garbage. It is also very dangerous! Who wants their spouse, a county health nurse, to make visits to crack cocaine houses and heroin shooting galleries? Who would volunteer to question these people about their needle sharing companions and bedroom partners?

Universal HIV screening would facilitate partner notification. Contact tracing would be made safer and much less expensive. The contacts will have already been tested as part of universal screening. No test—no driver's license. No test—no social security number. No test—no Medicare card. No test—no welfare check. No test—no citizenship. To control this epidemic we have *no choice*. It would matter less if person "o" acquired infection from person "x" "y" or "z". That is information we do not know today, anyway. What would matter is that person "o" does not infect persons "a" "b" or "c", who are not yet infected.

Everyone HIV-positive must be identified, counseled, and monitored. Everyone means everyone. Only by controlling the epidemic can we avoid worsening social chaos. Controlling the epidemic is the only means to limit needless suffering and death. Controlling the epidemic will not come at the hands of a vaccine or miracle drug. Controlling the epidemic requires prevention. Prevention requires knowing who is communicable. Knowing who is communicable requires universal testing (testing everyone). This is the only course available. It is not pleasant for me to accept. I have listened to all the nonsense and excuses for the past 10 years, ever since the AIDS test was first made available in 1985. I even bought into some of the nonsense. Today I am totally convinced that universal testing is necessary and long overdue.

The cost of treating 4,000,000 Americans with AIDS, at $100,000 per year by the year 2002, comes to about $400,000,000,000 annually. What about the year 2003, 2004, and so on? We will run out of zeros before a single life is saved. Pain and suffering are already horrendous. Help from the outside won't be forthcoming. The rest of the world will be similarly devastated. Within 35 years everyone will either be in need of treatment or rendering treatment!

I vote we spend the $4.00 today. It's about what it costs to park your car in Manhattan for 20 minutes.

6,000 TIMES WORSE

28

More people will die this year in Zaire of AIDS than from all the recorded deaths over the past 30 years from Ebola. The story is no better for the rest of Africa.

HIV is to Ebola what a nuclear bomb is to a fire cracker. HIV is *horrible*. Ebola is only *miserable*. 1995 was one of the worst recorded years for Ebola. An individual had one chance in 30 million of dying from this virus. If one lived on the African continent the odds increased to one chance in 4 million. *For each person who died of Ebola in 1995, at least 6,000 people died of AIDS.*

HIV, Ebola, Marburg, and Lassa Fever are all deadly tropical viruses. If any of them should ever mutate by altering their mode of transmission, allowing for rapid person-to-person spread by simple *air-borne* route (similar to influenza virus), all efforts of containment would be futile.

In 1976 there were two Ebola virus outbreaks, one in Sudan and one in Zaire, carried by similar but distinct strains of virus. There was another sporadic case in Zaire in 1977 and another Sudan outbreak in 1979. There is retrospective evidence for another two Ebola cases in Zaire in 1972 when a young nursing student rapidly succumbed to this infection. A resident doctor who performed an autopsy on her became critically ill but survived. The gruesome events of disseminated intravascular coagulation (DIC) that these two people suffered was colorfully depicted in the book, *The Hot Zone.*

In 1989 an outbreak of Ebola virus occurred at the Reston Virginia Primate Quarantine Unit. There were many primate deaths, although no human-related illness despite frequent accidental and inadvertent exposures. The potential for a human outbreak did exist.

There are glaring clinical differences, discussed below, that distinguish the HIVirus from the Ebola virus. I assure you that HIVirus is the real monster!

The AIDS pandemic is unrelenting. Some describe this ongoing global epidemic as now being in a broad second wave of destruction, superimposed upon an earlier, more selective wave of death. The first wave primarily targeted gay men, IV drug abusers, hemophiliacs, and heterosexuals in sub-Saharan Africa. **The second wave includes you and everyone you know.** HIVirus has already killed millions of human beings. Many more are currently HIV-infected and will certainly die. Millions of others who are not yet infected will become infected and will also die. In contrast, Ebola has killed relatively few humans, but those who die do so rapidly and dramatically—Hollywood style.

In March–April 1995, a serious outbreak of Ebola took place in the Rift Valley region of Zaire, with the epicenter at Kikwit City. Estimates are that 241 people died during the peak 4 weeks of this Ebola epidemic. Death came swiftly to these people. An area with a population of over 600,000 was quarantined. The ill were quickly identified and further isolated within the quarantine zone. The world applauded this great feat of public health. On the other hand, AIDS continually runs rampant in Zaire, threatening the entire population. Estimates are that 100 to 500 people acquire HIV *daily* in this sub-Saharan nation. Even in the midst of the recent Ebola outbreak in Zaire, it is certain that many more people in that nation acquired HIV (and will die of AIDS) than actually died of Ebola. The Ebola outbreak was contained-the death rate returned to zero. HIV and its destruction marches on.

One can only wonder what would have happened in Zaire if the choice had been made to contain Ebola only by education and not by enforcing sound public health policy. In contrast to Ebola, there are usually no initial symptoms to identify AIDS. By dismissing the practice of public health, the HIV-infected individual may not be identified until many years later. During this interval of time this person is usually feeling healthy but likely to be spreading infection. The large *unidentified* population of HIV-contagious individuals makes it impossible to contain the AIDS epidemic. The choice has been made to contain Ebola but not AIDS!

Those acutely infected with Ebola are contagious—the reason for quarantine. There is only a short interval during which there is person-to-person spread of Ebola (or measles or chicken pox for that matter). The survivors of Ebola are neither chronically infected nor chronically contagious. Outside a brief window of time, when the Ebola virus can rarely be recovered from semen or liver specimens, there are generally no persistent infectious particles in bodily secretions. Since there is no prolonged carrier state for Ebola, any epidemic like AIDS is much less likely to occur. In contrast to Ebola, everyone infected with HIVirus is a chronic carrier and remains contagious for life.

Not everyone infected with the Ebola virus becomes critically ill. One recent study points out that small children seem to be relatively spared of clinical disease. In parts of Zaire there is moderate prevalence of Ebola virus antibody (9%) detected in random blood specimens, yet few people with disease. This suggests the Ebola virus might be less virulent than was originally thought, causing many mild or subclinical cases. By contrast, almost everyone infected with HIV eventually becomes critically ill. I suspect that many of the survivors of Ebola will someday become infected with HIV and die of AIDS.

Humans are capable of mounting a protective immune

response to Ebola. People who survive Ebola illness develop antibodies. There are no reported recurrences of infection in survivors. This suggests that there would be a reasonable possibility of developing a vaccine against the Ebola virus should it ever be necessary. In contrast, a protective neutralizing antibody response does not occur against the HIVirus. Therefore, the prospect of developing an AIDS vaccine looks very grim.

No one has ever died of Ebola in the United States. If this should ever occur, it would be far easier to contain than HIV. It is astounding how fearful the Western world has become of Ebola and how accepting it has become of AIDS. If the media has frightened you about Ebola, then HIV should freeze your blood. I am frequently questioned about what the US government would do if Ebola should ever surface here. Ironically, so few people seem to care about what our government is not doing now, while HIV is already here, and here to stay.

AIDS is a disease with a mortality approaching 100%. Once serious symptoms develop they are unrelenting. No one with AIDS gets sick, recovers, and then lives on happily ever after. Everyone dies! Millions of people have already been lost to the AIDS holocaust. Nearly everyone infected with HIV in the 1970's has died. Most of the people infected with HIV in the 1980's are dead, dying, or ill. Those infected today will suffer the same fate.

Will the *real OUTBREAK* please stand up?

N B AIDS

29

Facts do not cease to exist because they are ignored.
— *Aldous Huxley*

He stands 6 feet 9 inches tall and weighs 256 pounds. When he speaks people listen. Karl Malone plays power forward for the Utah Jazz of the National Basketball Association (NBA). Into the early part of the 1991–92 season he and several other players threatened not to play in any games where there was a perceived threat of HIV exposure. The war cry, "I love this game!" was being challenged. This situation surfaced after basketball star Earvin "Magic" Johnson was injured and bled during a game. Magic had publicly acknowledged his HIV status during the off season.

Stunned and dumbfounded by Magic's announcement, Americans were certain that *now* they would have to find a cure. Heroes aren't supposed to die! The public confused scientific magic with Earvin Magic. Pressured not to play by other players around the league, the great career of a great athlete came to an apparent end. He had no symptoms. His decision was courageous. His illness was contagious—but was it on the court? He left the sport he loved and the sport that loved him. At the time of his departure from basketball he was the all-time player in assists. Magic left behind many other records and memories, not the least of which is that he is the first international athlete to leave a sport because of an HIV diagnosis.

Responsible leadership that reinforces the message of *prevention* will do more to help in the battle against AIDS than AZT, 3TC, and all the rest of the superstar drugs (that don't cure anybody) combined. It is now HIV clutch-time. At stake is something more precious than an NBA championship ring—it is the health of our children. For each adolescent who will become a professional athlete, thousands will become HIV-infected. Some will become both. I believe Magic's greatest assist is yet to come.

The actual risk of transmitting AIDS while competing on the basketball court, football field, or in a swimming pool is not known. The unknown hazard at the professional level is likewise ill-defined at the college level, in high school, and on the playground. The variable risk factors include how many people are infected, the types of exposures encountered, and what precautions might be taken.

Communicable diseases are described in association with sports. These predominately include infections that are spread air-borne such as influenza and pertussis. Also included are chickenpox, measles, and other nonblood-borne pathogens. Herpes gladiatorum can occur in outbreaks among wrestlers. This is caused by skin-to-skin contact of herpes simplex virus.

Historically, blood-borne diseases such as hepatitis B have only rarely been transmitted through contact sports. There is a report of Japanese sumo wrestlers who acquired hepatitis B as a consequence of that sport. Swedish athletes engaging in another sport known as orienteering (track-finding in the wilderness), have spread hepatitis B by blood contact with other competitors.

A report from Varese, Italy, describes the transmission of HIVirus to a 25 year-old man who collided with another player during a soccer match. The collision caused both players to sustain severe facial skin injuries with copious bleeding. Some players on one team were known to be drug abusers. The suspected drug-abusing player involved in the collision was HIV-positive. The other player, who had previously tested HIV-negative, and had no other risk factors, developed a mild mononucleosis-like syndrome one month later. Two months after the incident he converted his HIV test to seropositive. He became infected.

Unlike the lurking danger that may be associated with dental procedures, I believe the transmission of HIVirus on the basketball court is presently very low. Because there is no universal screening, I don't know just how low. HIV transmission has been reported as a consequence of bite injuries and bloody fights. Health care workers have acquired HIVirus through occupational exposure. Most of these cases were caused by needle-stick injuries. At least seven separate cases, and I suspect several more, occurred as a direct complication of blood-splash injury to the face. This same blood contact scenario would present risk to athletes if other athletes were infected. However, in the larger picture of this epidemic, this type of transmission is minimal. The best way to avoid this accidental exposure is to control the epidemic outside the sporting arena. An athlete who is infected is far more likely to spread the virus in nonsporting activities (unless one considers sex or intravenous drug abuse a sport).

Spectators have also been known to receive injuries. *Bloody* European soccer brawls involving fans have disrupted games. National news highlighted a spectator head injury at a golf tournament in Palm Desert, California. The stray golf ball was stroked by former President George Bush. It is doubtful that any tournament officials came prepared with rubber gloves or level 4 biosafety suits.

What is alarming is that more people today are HIV-infected than ever before. This includes athletes as well as everyone else. Any inadvertent blood exposure today carries a higher risk than any similar exposure to blood in the past. The risk of acquiring AIDS in competitive sports is somewhere above zero, but relatively low. This risk will increase with time.

Does banning an HIV-positive athlete from participating in sports also mean he/she should be banned from driving a car? Might not this same athlete be injured elsewhere and present risk to others? And what about everyone else? Does the potential for an accident suggest a driver's license be revoked if the driver is HIV-positive? Or what about just being a passenger? Accidents happen all the time. Why should sports receive exclusive attention? Certain risks are unavoidable. What is important is that the epidemic be controlled with attention focused on everyone equally. What is important is that the epidemic be controlled!

There will always be inadvertent blood exposures. The average human carries approximately nine pints of blood at any one time. A single infected individual harbors a viral population 10 times greater than the entire human population. How are we to be protected from blood exposures associated with vehicle accidents, natural disasters, terrorists attacks, and playground nose bleeds?

A zero risk environment is not achievable, but we can minimize danger. As a greater percentage of the population becomes HIV-infected so will more athletes. As the epidemic grows there will also be more people infected without symptoms. If there is no mandatory screening, most of those infected will remain unaware of their status until years later, when illness strikes. The only way to lower the risk of HIV exposure resulting from competitive sports is to control the epidemic in the general population. This requires prevention where the risk is greatest: sexual exposure, intravenous drug abuse, bodily fluid exposure, and newborn transmission.

HIV antibody screening has dramatically reduced the risk associated with blood product transfusion, tissue transplants, and sperm donations. Properly applied, universal screening (everyone) along with public health intervention are our best defensive weapons against HIVirus. Estimates are that over half of the HIV-positive population, athletes included, have never even been tested. Since when is an untested HIV-positive athlete safer than a tested HIV-positive athlete? If it is considered unsafe for Magic Johnson to play basketball, then it should also be considered unsafe for any athlete who does not know his or her HIV status (and may be contagious) to play basketball. What applies to Madison Square Garden or to the Forum should also apply to the playground.

Olympic diver, Greg Louganis, meant no harm to come from an unexpected head injury that spilled HIV-infected blood into the Olympic pool in Seoul, South Korea. The risk to other divers was probably negligible. The risk to the team physician who sutured Louganis's scalp at poolside without gloves was not! The poor surgical hygiene used was potentially a death sentence for this physician. The HIV status of anyone, athlete or not, should be made perfectly clear to any health care provider or Good Samaritan. One obvious way to make this possible is to get tested and to provide this information.

Basketball is not boxing—ice hockey, I'm not so sure about. Only in professional boxing and in the martial arts is there any attempt to implement HIV screening in sports. As of early 1996, Oregon, Washington, Arizona, and Nevada were the only states that required testing of boxers. Boxing is a blood-letting sport. The risk of blood-splash injuries in boxing is significant, especially when both opponents have multiple open wounds. When and if testing is required of all boxers, more HIV infections will be identified. The risk of an infected boxer passing the HIVirus to another boxer in the ring (or to a lover in bed) is real.

When heavyweight boxer Tommy Morrison tested HIV-positive he was banned from the sport. This may have saved other boxers the agony of HIV infection. The awareness of his positive HIV status may have also saved the lives of those he cares about outside the ring. The courage of Tommy Morrison to publicly acknowledge his HIV infection and the impact it may have on others prompted New York and several other states to reevaluate HIV testing in athletics. All boxers should be HIV tested and all boxers testing positive should be restricted from that sport. It was good fortune that Tommy Morrison was scheduled to compete in Las Vegas, Nevada, where testing of boxers is mandatory. Otherwise, his silent HIV status might not have been revealed to him. His contacts can now be protected (hopefully it is not too late). The fight Morrison must now champion is bigger than a personal boxing title; it is to help the world defeat a heavyweight virus. Legislation mandating HIV testing must be enacted for boxers and nonboxers. Smelling salts are needed for the forty-six states without mandatory HIV testing of boxers—and for the fifty states without mandatory testing of everyone!

I applaud Greg Louganis's courage when he recently shared with the world his own personal tragedy. During a public interview with Barbara Walters, Louganis implored that all HIV-positive people be more responsible. That responsibility must include doing everything necessary to avoid spreading this infection to anyone else. Once infected there is no way to get uninfected. Drugs and vaccines don't give you a second chance. A billion dollars cannot buy you out of this one. An untold number of people around the world are learning this lesson. They are either dead, dying, soon to be ill, or soon to be infected!

Man is pushed up against the ropes. This virus does not look for a first round knockout. It is always satisfied with the unanimous decision. It wants to fight 12 rounds (years), taking on countless new victims in the same fight. Education is just a cornerman—it doesn't put on the gloves. **We are the ones in the ring!**

EVERY THIRTEEN MONTHS

30

Not all microorganisms are *created equal!* The AIDS community has been *dying* under a gross misconception. The public has been *living* under a gross misconception. These errors were born of hope and desperation, not of deceit. No one is to blame. **A virus is no bacteria.**

Seemingly good news might turn bad. Word from Europe in late 1983 was that the French had recovered a lenti-type retrovirus from a lymph node of an AIDS patient. It was called LAV (Lymphadenopathy Associated Virus). I remember the feeling of shared hope that a discovery may have been made. By this time reports were already circulating that the number of new cases of AIDS in America was doubling every thirteen months. Most victims were gay men living in urban centers. We needed to hear some good news. Curiosity about an unusual but deadly disease was turning to panic.

Today many of these same urban areas are reporting 50% saturation of HIVirus in members of the gay community *still alive.* Each death is replaced by several new infections. In the game of AIDS statistics you are counted out when you are counted dead.

By 1984 American investigators at the NIH (National Institutes of Health) confirmed the findings of the French that HTLV III (Human T-cell Lymphoma Virus) and LAV were the same virus. By joint agreement in 1985, HIV became the designated name for this newly discovered virus. The key word is **virus.**

A cure was expected. After all, this is the assumed job of science. Science cured The Plague and eradicated smallpox. Why should this be different?

I remember my apprehension at the time. I had treated multitudes of serious bacterial infections, almost always with good results. Viral infections could not be treated the same way; they could only be prevented. This required the public health measures of isolation and immunization. When confronted with viral infections the only effective therapy was treating symptoms while the body fought off the virus. We did not have drugs that eradicated any virus. We still don't. This point was ignored; it remains ignored. **A virus is no bacteria.**

Intelligent, gifted people were dropping dead. Something had to be done. Never mind it was a *virus,* something had to be done. In 1985 little was known about the natural course of this disease. Very few would have believed that there would be an 8 to 10 year incubation period from the time of initial exposure to the development of symptoms. No one comprehended what implications this would have for the development of a vaccine. If a person was infected with the live natural virus, and after so many years could still not develop protective immunity, what hope would there be for an effective vaccine. With every viral infection known to mankind, the best vaccine is always the natural infection. Pertaining to AIDS, this best vaccine, the live natural virus, is a complete flop.

This is the **brick wall** that activists and all concerned are trying to walk through. The *virus* is what lies behind the misconception. **A virus is no bacteria.** There is not a single drug that eliminates any virus, HIVirus being no exception. This is a smart virus. It does not behave in such a way that it allows the human body to develop effective neutralizing antibodies. This makes the possibility of a vaccine remote. It is time we get smart too. Our only hope is to prevent transmission. We continue to ignore and obstruct the obvious.

This clever virus graduated at the top of its class. It is a formidable foe. It captures you first, then silently destroys your defenses. Not until the end does it finally declare war. No hostage survives. This virus can only be challenged *before* the initial exposure. Scientists, health care providers, and activists miss this simple truth.

ACT-UP (AIDS Coalition To Unleash Power) is one group that was founded as a response to what was *not* happening, foremost, a cure. The death toll was mounting, consisting primarily of gay men. Did the government not care? Who would protect privacy, civil rights, jobs, and insurance coverage? Where are the pharmaceutical giants? Unleash power! Attract attention! Now! Never mind the disruption of an International AIDS Conference, a religious service, or a health department meeting. No one cares! We are dying! Hard to disagree with. Hardly a solution.

The path to hell is paved with good intentions. Enlightened, socially responsible citizens are reacting to the AIDS crisis. The heart and soul of all efforts put into education remain unrewarded. The gay community has attempted to demonstrate leadership, but in the meantime, its membership is being cruelly defined by the AIDS epidemic. We have all miscalculated the significance that **a virus is no bacteria.**

There is no cure for AIDS and there may never be. Are we waiting for divine intervention? Epidemiology with a beating pulse is imperative. Identification and contact tracing is an integral part of prevention. No policy should ever derail prevention. No organization, public or private, gay or straight, should obstruct universal testing and necessary intervention. The protection of privacy and civil rights, which I support, must be adjusted to accommodate the overriding necessity to contain this epidemic.

The danger of individual abuse of personal freedom is real. Examples make the headlines everyday. The abuse of personal freedom is now fueling the AIDS epidemic into today's tragic reality. From the Palais Des Congres to the halls of the FDA, echo the desperate chants, "AIDS treatment now, Illness is Death! We've got it! AIDS action now!" I ask, what about the call for responsibility and prevention now? If someone weighs 450 pounds, it is bad for their health. If they sit on you, it is bad for your health.

From the bedside of a person with AIDS, the pleading cry continues, "Release the drugs!" The drugs have been released and they have not worked. More drugs will be released and they will likely be just as worthless. **A virus is no bacteria.** On deck are the protease inhibitors. They also will not save a single person. Let us pray I am wrong.

"Silence is death," drones the next mantra demanding a cure. The message should be that HIV is an incurable virus and ignoring this truth is death. The world does not need ACT-UPS (AIDS Coalition to Undermine Public Safety). The world needs a revitalized and compassionate ACT-UP (AIDS Coalition to Unleash Power) that understands that *power is in prevention.* Disregarding public safety, avoiding personal responsibility, and not accepting behavioral change will guarantee death. ACT-UP and similar groups have an important role to play. I hope they discover this role.

We can blame Ronald, George or Bill. Government has no answer. No government can cure earthquakes. Don't waste time insisting they can. Governments must respond when an earthquake occurs. Make sure they do. AIDS is the earthquake that won't quit shaking!

The strongest swimmer, swimming in circles, will eventually drown. Every eight minutes in this country someone new becomes infected, taking the plunge. They will drown. A scream for a rescue must be echoed by a scream for prevention. Sharing the responsibility of monitoring responsible behavior, the gay community needs to be poised to lead the charge demanding universal testing and intervention. It must be guaranteed that everyone who may have been exposed be notified and that everyone who is infected be counseled for life. Demand the right to participate, not just the right to complain. It is a matter of survival for the gay community. It is a matter of survival for everyone.

Our first identification must be with the human species. The world suffers miserably when people identify primarily with their race, religion or nationality. Today we also suffer because sexual preference has found its way to the top of this list.

ON SANTA'S LAP

Oh, you can get it if you really want.
—Jimmy Cliff

31

Jeffrey was sobbing uncontrollably in the scorching heat. We had just lowered Dean into the ground. He was crouched over the gravesite.

I was honored to have been asked to be a pallbearer, but I was also in a hurry and needed to leave. I had hospital patients to visit on medical rounds. I knew I would see Jeffrey again.

Both men had recently moved to Ojai, California. They set up business in their new home as interior designers. They had a number of clients in the area and decided this foothill community with oak trees and art galleries was just what they were looking for. No doubt they would have enjoyed living in Ojai had they been well and lived longer.

Dean was already quite ill when we first met. He had severe weight loss, uncontrolled diarrhea, and a painful neuropathy that left him with shooting sensations down both legs. He could walk only with assistance. He swore never to be hospitalized, and he wasn't. He died in his new home shortly after we met.

Jeffrey was not as symptomatic. He mentioned

occasional night sweats, but otherwise felt well. I saw him more in the context of caring for Dean through his terminal event.

I had occasion to be at a medical conference in San Francisco the week before Christmas of that year. My family was with me. I had never been to Macy's Department Store at Christmas. My wife thought it would be fun for our kids to see the decorations and meet Santa. The store was mobbed. The holiday spirit was captured with an array of decorative displays.

Waiting in "Santa Claus Lane," my son was excitedly about to plop onto the lap of the bearded old man. My eyes caught a glimpse of a couple standing in the next aisle over. There was Jeffrey, his arms around a young man I had never seen before. Dean had died about four months earlier. Normally I would have been glad to see Jeffrey, but just then I didn't feel that way. My immediate thought was, "How could he?" Dean was already dead, but was Jeffrey being unfaithful to this young man around whose waist his arm was now wrapped? Did this young man know he was in trouble? He was either infected or about to become infected. By then we knew how AIDS was transmitted and who was dying. So did Jeffrey.

Jeffrey never came back to see me. I learned a year later that he had died elsewhere of an AIDS-associated cancer. I know nothing about the young man Jeffrey was embracing at Macy's during that joyous holiday season.

The picture of my son, Rhett, innocently sitting on Santa's lap, remains fresh in my mind.

HEALER OR ACCOMPLICE?

*The man who regards his own life
and that of his fellow creatures
as meaningless is not merely
unhappy but hardly fit for life.*
— *Albert Einstein*

32

CAUTION! Do not include this chapter. . . .
Activists will go berserk. . . . It is hardball
bigotry. . . . It will be misunderstood!

I believe reasonable people will understand
and welcome all dialogue. This chapter is part of
the story of this epidemic.

Many different drugs have been tried for the
purpose of keeping AIDS patients alive. Results
are temporary. Some patients live longer because
of improved treatment against opportunistic
infections. Drugs that are directly targeted against
the HIVirus, in my opinion, have not made a
significant difference. I do not believe that newer
drugs, used in combination, will be the
revolutionary breakthrough everyone is hoping
for. I would like to be wrong.

AIDS patients must be counseled. They hold
the key to controlling this epidemic. I always
request that family or partners be involved in this
process. This is welcomed by most patients. I
believe physicians must play a proactive and
responsible role in the lives of patients who are
capable of doing grave harm to others—so should
public health officials. I also believe most patients

accept more personal responsibility for their behavior when engaged in closer counseling. Many HIV-infected people, heterosexual and homosexual, do not behave responsibly. While being kept alive many are spreading this virus—while awaiting their own death, they spread death. Every person infected was infected by someone else. Almost every gay man who died of AIDS in the last fifteen years was infected by another gay man. This _truth_ merits open discussion.

I will never forget one particular patient. David, a fictitious first name, is a very real person. I was the fourth Infectious Disease specialist he had seen for his AIDS-related ailments. I knew I would not be the last. On his third visit to see me he complained of a penile discharge. Gonorrhea. He boasted of a weekend escapade to Palm Springs. I questioned whether he had informed sexual contacts of his HIV status. In no uncertain terms and in a memorably loud shriek, the reprimand came, "My business is none of your business. Who are you to invade my privacy?"

California law (section 11166 of the penal code) dictates that any physician who is even suspicious of child abuse must make an immediate report to authorities. Failure to do so can result in serious fines. If an HIV-infected patient is knowingly spreading a deadly virus, physicians are petrified to say anything. We know exactly what is happening, but not to _whom_ it is happening. We do nothing! We are afraid of the legal consequences. So are the people who are responsible for tracing contacts.

Was I the mechanic repairing David's car, knowing he would use his vehicle to run over your son or daughter? Would this make me an accomplice? What is the responsibility physicians have to public safety? Is the Hippocratic Oath so sacred to the patients we treat that it is now treacherous to the society in which we live? This man, a computer engineer with no criminal record, showed no sense of remorse.

For years I have been haunted by this person. The law is on his side. Common sense is ignored. Morality is faltering. The virus is spreading. More people are dying.

Attempts are being made to sustain the lives of those who

are HIV-infected. While being kept alive, no HIV-positive person has the right to infect and kill someone else with this disease. There is no dictum that gives anyone the right to take another life through careless behavior. This is the paramount reason why everyone must know if he or she is infected, to avoid inadvertently killing others. Is that too much to ask?

Punishment is not the question here—responsible behavior is. There is no way to reverse an individual tragedy. Prevention is possible. Cure is beyond our grasp. Society deserves the safeguard that no infected person will spread this virus. Education alone is without teeth. Each infection is everyone's business. **Civil liberties will need to be redefined.**

LITIGAIDS:
The Right To Be Dead Right!

33

Row upon serried row they sit, all experts to the rule.
But there is only one, my friend, who must fight the bull.
— Garcia Lorca (revised)

Philadelphia is America's symbolic City of Brotherly Love. The Declaration of Independence, the Liberty Bell, and now the movie. The new rallying cry for change, "Philadelphia." Now they'll listen. Now they'll hear the truth. Hollywood is finally getting involved. At last!

What went wrong? Don't Oscars count? Why aren't *they* doing something now? Is there no *they*, like there is no *cure?* Could our best actors fail us?

The movie missed the picture. *Philadelphia* was well directed and well acted. Unfortunately, it was a triumph for the Legal Aids epidemic and not the AIDS epidemic. The adversarial agenda, rather than mutual cooperation, made it to the big screen. At last, popcorn, soda pop, and Legal AIDS. I believe the movie did more to encourage young people to become attorneys than AIDS researchers.

A stinging footnote, an American saga: it is reported that the family of the AIDS patient portrayed in *Philadelphia* has since been in litigation with the movie's producers!

The American legal system has discovered AIDS. Trouble! This may be the most dangerous discovery in world history.

AIDS does not belong in the court room! Thirty years ago AIDS would have been recognized as a medical condition, an infectious disease. Today it is recognized as a legal condition entangled in the conflict between individual rights and public safety. The epidemic should be managed by scientists, epidemiologists, physicians, nurses, and other health care professionals. Controlling transmission requires an informed and compassionate society. Twelve people in a box deliberating AIDS-related monetary awards is counter-productive. We must all comprise the jury. The only acceptable verdict is containing the epidemic!

Honor and goodwill have been abandoned. The life-blood of the legal profession is colored green. It is the profit made from conflict. AIDS is all about social conflict and medical failure. As such, it is a magnet for lawyers and litigation. There are no adequate standards of care. The treatment of each patient changes daily. Clinical outcome ranges from dismal to horrible. Most HIV infections conclude with death and there is always pain and suffering. Treatment by trial and error is a necessary component of therapy. *Guess who loves pain and suffering, trials and errors?*

Just as man seems to have no natural immunity to HIVirus, AIDS certainly has no immunity to lawyers. There is no shortage of legal AIDS facilitators. Might there be more legal AIDS clinics than medical AIDS clinics? At this moment more lawyers are contemplating how to litigate issues regarding this virus than there are scientists struggling with ways to eradicate it. Attorneys show more interest in the practice of legal AIDS than physicians show interest in the practice of treating AIDS. This is a sad testimonial to both professions.

I was recently paged by an AIDS patient. I had met this gentleman only once. He had not yet obtained the CD4 count I had ordered two weeks ago. He was requesting a recommendation for a "good HIV lawyer." He politely informed me he appreciated my help and would feel comfortable with the care I could give him. He would reschedule an appointment to see me after he obtained a lawyer. My comfort zone with him dropped to zero.

The University of California enrolls over 3,400 law students (1994 Fall headcount in the Juris Doctorate programs at Boalt, UCLA, Davis, and Hastings). Maintaining the four UC Law Schools is an annual expense to California tax payers of $35 million (excluding private funds and endowments)—not bad for a struggling California economy. Should any public law school falter, there are countless private law schools to keep the fire storm alive. Coincidentally, there is serious consideration for cutting funds for AIDS programs, closing busy public hospitals, and eliminating schools of nursing and public health. The same reason is consistently given—lack of funds. It's no secret that we are also losing the battle against AIDS. Dare we close the doors of a single law school!

The primary responsibility of public health services is to protect us when we are alive and well, not to count us when we are dying or dead. The legal hurdles of the AIDS epidemic are as formidable as the scientific hurdles. In order to properly inform and notify contacts of HIV, rights of privacy and confidentiality are unavoidably infringed upon. The very statutes that serve to protect individual rights are now legal barriers to the pragmatism necessary to halt the relentless spread of a fatal disease. The identification and notification process is a legal quagmire. The choice to preserve civil liberties to their extreme and to disregard public safety is today's choice between life and death. Let us stop being afraid to act. AIDS policy should always be formulated with a keen eye on the virus, not on lawyers.

"I want you to treat me, but I do not want anyone to recognize me in your waiting room. I do not want my diagnosis part of my medical record. Is that clear, doctor?" Assembly Bill 403 (AB403) became California law in 1985. Any California doctor who was unable to protect the privacy of an HIV patient or who felt the disclosure was in the public's interest could now be subjected to a $10,000 fine and one year of imprisonment per infraction. This threat would be spelled out in black and white. The law would not be amended until January, 1989. Similar laws were enacted in other states. Confidentiality would take precedence over therapy. **AIDS was officially declared a legal entity, not a communicable disease.**

An entire generation of physicians that might have more willingly cared for AIDS patients was wiped out by legal intimidation. They took cover. Few of my colleagues dared manage AIDS, even those patients from families they had known for years. The legal hazard was too threatening. Confusion over the preservation of confidentiality, and the never ending threat of litigation, interfere with patient care. Confidentiality is impossible to guarantee. How would it be possible to ensure that a laboratory or radiology technician would not recognize a certain name? For what other disease might a pharmacist think AZT is prescribed? For what other condition is aerosolized pentamidine used? It is impossible to hide this disease. AIDS identification is unmasked by physical appearance. A wasted-appearing 32 year-old male, with purple clusters dotting his forehead, is not dying from flea bites. AIDS is not a rare disease. AIDS is not a zebra on a surfboard.

Physicians are required to keep careful medical records. How, one might ask, is it possible to keep accurate records of a patient with AIDS and not mention the diagnosis of AIDS or HIV on the medical chart? Patients may request (or the law might require) that an AIDS diagnosis not be revealed when medical records are requested or subpoenaed. Physicians are supposed to doctor patients, not doctor charts. Health care providers intimidated by such twisted confidentiality statutes frequently chose not to treat AIDS patients. I know, they refer them to me or to other Infectious Disease specialists. All too often I hear the concern, "I don't understand the meaning of all the laws and rules." No one does. On balance, the liability fears associated with maintenance of privacy do patients far more harm than good. A grave error is being made by trying to control the AIDS epidemic by hiding its casualties.

Coast to coast, every state is buried with conflicting legal statutes. Physicians now attend conferences aboard cruise ships and at ski resorts to learn about the newest AIDS laws. Continuing medical education (CME) credits are offered to be a *legal* AIDS expert. No lives are saved by this. The only thing protected is the skin of doctors. The educational time would be more valuable if focused on how better to treat AIDS, rather than on how to be protected against AIDS litigation. In fact, it would be much better just to go skiing!

The most effective AIDS care is individualized treatment. No two patients are in the same stage of disease. Expectations and attitudes are completely variable and change as the disease progresses. The response and tolerance to medications vary. There may be significant genetic differences among hosts as well as differences in the virulence of the virus. The same opportunistic infections affect each person with different severity. Some patients prefer an active role in all therapeutic decisions. Other patients opt for their physicians to manage everything.

Standardized care is not appropriate in the treatment of AIDS. Guidelines are useful as long as they are flexible. Physicians are accustomed to the concept of "standard of care." This is an influence of the legal profession, not a consequence of proper medical training. Attorneys thrive on any deviation from the "standard of care" concept. AIDS is easy fodder for litigation.

All of us are (or should be) AIDS-phobic, homosexuals included. No one wants to contract any dreaded disease that has no cure and has already claimed millions of lives. AIDS initially exploded in the gay population, a medical fact that cannot be erased. While homophobia continues to exist, it should not be mistaken for AIDS-phobia. Every surgeon I know would rather operate on an HIV-negative homosexual than a HIV-positive heterosexual. Many health care providers have already been infected as a consequence of their profession. The fear of AIDS overshadows the fear of someone else's sexual preference. The real winner of the phobia lineup is legal-phobia. It interferes with the willingness of health care providers to even become involved with those who are infected and need their help.

The burden of litigation is *not* just about AIDS; it is about America. It is about employee against employer, patient against doctor, neighbor against neighbor, lover against lover. What have we become? We find ourselves adversaries, alienated and alone. People with AIDS experience the brunt of this. 300 million people are no longer connected—the stars and stripes are tearing apart.

It is always better to sacrifice confidentiality than human lives. Public health officers cannot notify every possible contact of an infected individual without infringement of privacy. Be reminded, these are the contacts of a fatal disease. These contacts will further spread this deadly virus. Over-notification is better than no notification. Honest mistakes and misunderstandings will occur. Public health officials are well aware of the conflict between individual rights and society's right to be protected. Too often, these same officials, whose job it is to protect the public safety, remain paralyzed in their public health responsibilities by legal intimidation. This intimidation has become accepted in this country as part of the social norm. This is not healthy. We adjust our behavior according to legal considerations—not according to what is right or wrong. The fear of litigation has become its own disease. Tragically, we are now accepting HIV as part of the norm in America as well.

I participate on AIDS advisory panels. Despite attendance by people with the best of intentions, nothing constructive is accomplished at most of these meetings. Certainly, no lives are saved. I believe my time is usually wasted. Other physicians share in this despair. Legal concerns factor heavily, if not entirely, in decision making. Policies are drafted with the first priority being to keep the draftees out of legal hot water. Always overshadowed is the original intent of the group, to stop the carnage of a deadly virus. No rule or law will ever do what humans themselves must do to confront the spread of this virus.

Throughout America health officials and AIDS advisors are busy adjusting AIDS policy—committees, subcommittees, sub-subcommittees. Meetings and memos are easy. The difficult field work, to trace contacts, is left unattended. The legal ramifications can be hazardous to your health.

Desperately needed are concerned public health officials who want to accept authority and responsibility and are willing to *make the necessary legal blunders to save lives.*

When a new case of AIDS is identified, county health departments *may* choose to investigate and notify possible contacts. The process is usually done anonymously, if at all. The health department caller is frequently not even identified. The exposed individual receives a phone message warning, "You may have been exposed to someone carrying the HIVirus." A spouse may be given no more information beyond a possible exposure warning. What health officials are really saying is, "We would like to help you but we do not wish to get ourselves in trouble." Stated more bluntly, "It is wiser for us to avoid a lawsuit than for you to avoid AIDS." Names are often not given for fear of litigation. In New York City it was policy that even mothers of HIV-positive newborn babies were not immediately informed of the child's status. It would interfere with the mother's privacy right *not* to know her own HIV status. Even John Lennon could not have *imagined* that one!

An individual who tests positive (100% contagious), and who has not met an arbitrary CDC categorization of AIDS, goes unreported. There is no contact tracing or partner notification. 50–70% of all Americans who are HIV-positive have never even been tested! This is the *deadliest* group. This has also been the easiest category for health officials to respond to—they don't respond at all!

Three years ago I attended a benefit gala for AIDS education. The stars were out that night. A young lady who identified herself as a public health official commented to our group, "We can't be held responsible when we don't know who is HIV-positive. It protects *us* that way." I remember the jolt I felt by her remark. This irresponsible attitude has never before existed in public health service. The twisted thinking indicated to me a greater fear of lawyers than of the HIVirus. Health officials were opting to tiptoe with blinders, preferring to avoid lawsuits than to uncover new cases of AIDS. I don't know how much money was raised that night, but I left wondering who needed to be educated.

In June, 1995, film actor Hugh Grant was arrested for alleged lewd conduct. The press was in a frenzy. At the time it was a commercial break of sorts for the O.J. Simpson Trial. The news was not really about what had occurred, but about who was involved. There are countless daily occurrences involving prostitution which elicit no attention. This one involved sex and stardom. Suddenly it became America's business.

It was decided that if Hugh Grant was convicted, "Not only would there *not* be an AIDS test, it would be prohibited for a judge to order one because of state privacy laws." This was the official comment from the city attorney's office. A *Los Angeles Times* article further explained that if convicted Grant would still be required to take an AIDS education class. One must then question, in the unfortunate event that he or anyone else was infected, would an educational class guarantee protection of any future contacts? Will education alone tell him or his partners whether they are already infected and need to seek medical help as soon as possible? Education should be conducted in conjunction with mandatory screening and ongoing counseling. Are we protecting the law or the virus? We should be protecting Mr. Grant and his contacts! No one deserves to die because of privacy laws.

Regarding AIDS, there should be but one law—**it is immoral to spread this virus under any circumstance.** This law should be universal. It should not have to require legislative process to enact or a judge to enforce. It must be on the conscience of every human being.

In late 1986 New York health officials realized they had a sticky problem on their hands. AIDS was being acquired by artificial sperm insemination. How could these entrusted health officials not realize that *the inseminated women who became HIV-infected were the ones who had the real problem?* A significant number of semen donors at commercial sperm banks were homosexual. Identification of some cases of HIV in recipients of donated sperm should have prompted immediate notification of all other women who were at risk from artificial insemination. The reluctance to participate in this "call back" stems from fear of liability. "We must protect the privacy of the donor," so they had been taught to think. Public health officials recognized the liability risks of contacting other recipients of HIV-infected sperm, as well as the additional contacts of those recipients, and so on. A legal nightmare could result from the wrong people inadvertently being notified. Similarly, physicians also wanted nothing to do with disclosing to sperm recipients that they may have been exposed to HIVirus at the doctor's facility—that death certificates for the mother and child might soon accompany the birth certificate! What was really protected was the right of this virus to infect new hosts. By 1989, four years after HIV testing was first made available, New York State finally enacted regulations to test organ and sperm donors. Mazel Tov!

How did we arrive at such legal excrement? Why has public safety been so severely compromised by the fear of litigation? Where are the safeguards to protect the uninfected? Why has there been no fight and so little discussion? Where has organized medicine been hiding? **Are doctors so preoccupied with health insurance that they have forgotten health?**

The HIV infection rate is rapidly climbing, interrupted only by death, not by cure. Epidemics must be managed by experienced epidemiologists working in cooperation with health care providers. Sound principles must be adhered to. AIDS is no exception. What we are experiencing in public health is a "no look, no see, no do" policy of default; a true public health meltdown. What is politically and legally safe for health officials is deadly for the population. Those who are responsible for protecting have decided to first protect themselves. Lawyers, bureaucrats, and special interest groups must step aside. Time is running out. **Having no cure and no vaccine, it is intolerable to have no prevention!**

The first stage of this epidemic has passed. It appears the only survivors will be those who remain uninfected. The HIVs and HIV-Nots must coexist. The sanctity of life can never be preserved in walled-off communities. Public health must serve the needs of all individuals, those infected and those who are not. We must safeguard the quality of life of those who are already infected. On that account we have not done well. This is more reason to safeguard against further massive spread of infection. It is unlikely that anyone infected in the future will do much better than those who are infected today. As more people become infected, more resources become depleted. As more people become infected, preventing spread will become much more difficult. A point is reached beyond which there is no cure, no vaccine, and no hope of containment.

Any carefully worked out AIDS screening policy will undoubtedly be held hostage by our current laws. Ironically, we now need our government to protect us from ourselves, from our own laws, and from our own lawyers. How does a society correct a legal system that ignores the general welfare for greed and profit? Under the false pretense of protecting civil liberties, Americans have actually seen freedoms diminish. No longer do we have the liberty to walk safely down any street. Many no longer feel safe in their homes. Is there a right not to get infected with a deadly virus?

The Second Amendment to the Constitution protects the right to bear arms. Does this include the right to infect another human being with a deadly virus? *Do we now have the right to be dead right?*

Some hold that common sense is now dead in America, suffocated by laws. If common sense is not dead, it is certainly struggling to be heard. The legal erosion of common sense extends deep into our ability to provide quality health care. Physicians must assert themselves as leaders of health care and force change in our legal system. I believe this action is ethical and responsible. Perhaps it is wishful thinking, but a litigation-free AIDS policy might spread an idea that deserves attention elsewhere in our legally strangulated society. Less litigation could also do wonders for the mental health of this nation!

There is a fine line between personal rights and public safety. A small retrovirus, about 90 nanometers in size, invisible to the naked eye and even to a high-powered microscope, now straddles that line. In this tug-of-war, people are walking wounded and dying in large numbers. A draconian change in our legal and public health systems is necessary to prevent further carnage.

Terminating the litigation epidemic is necessary before we can control the AIDS epidemic!

PIN THE DONKEY ON THE TAIL

34

D eath passes person-to-person. As in child's play, we are blindfolded. But by whose choice?

Twenty years ago a homeless person in America stood out. Today millions of homeless are part of the American landscape. They are barely noticed. Violent crime, once abhorred, has gained acceptance as part of our culture. AIDS has taken a similar path. At one time a medical curiosity, AIDS is now the leading killer of middle-aged men. Women are catching up. We are awash in complacency.

Many of those who die of AIDS have no idea who slipped them the lethal pathogen. The indelible trail of death remains uninterrupted. The scorekeepers at public health monitor death but do little to preserve life. There is no precedent in medical history where a concerted effort is made *not* to know who is infected with a lethal, communicable disease. The institutions responsible for safeguarding public welfare are boxseat spectators. The ability to test and intervene has now been available for over eleven years. The only mandatory application of HIV screening has been for blood and tissue products. This has saved many lives. It came too late for the hemophiliac population, which has been decimated by AIDS. Even the obvious application of screening by blood banks did not come without a fight from activists.

Universal testing opens the door to early intervention. Included is better control of opportunistic infections and AIDS-related tumors. Some investigators now suggest that if antiretroviral treatment is of any benefit, it should be initiated as soon as possible after exposure.

Universal testing would help better define risk factors of transmission.

Universal testing would allow the identification of non-progressors who could be carefully evaluated. The knowledge gained might give insight into vaccine development.

Universal testing would identify nearly everyone who is positive. Most people who are positive at this moment have never been tested or informed. There is a short window period after exposure when testing cannot yet detect seroconversion. Improved technology can narrow this period and repeat testing would allow identification of those hidden within the window period.

Universal testing would allow for focused education and direct counseling to everyone infected.

Universal testing would permit responsible public health intervention regarding irresponsible behavior that jeopardizes the safety of others, i.e. the lives of others.

Universal testing would ease the burden and cost of contact notification. Secondary and tertiary cases would automatically be identified if universal screening was initiated.

Universal testing would reduce unnecessary surgical and dental risks.

Universal testing, by identifying unsuspected cases, would clarify our knowledge about safe sex. One may wisely choose no sex over safe sex when the HIV status of a partner is known to be positive.

Universal testing would give early warning to other associated infectious diseases such as tuberculosis. Controlling the tuberculosis epidemic now requires controlling the AIDS epidemic.

Universal testing is a public health measure, not a punitive reaction. It should signal to young people that society cares about their well being. Every effort must be made to protect against a disease for which there is no cure. Infection control is *not* about stripping away rights, it is about keeping people alive and healthy. The best way to maintain privacy is to not expose oneself to this deadly virus. Your privacy is compromised when you get sick.

Universal testing would bring truth to HIV statistics. Each HIV statistic is an HIV casualty. We need to know where we are. Are there 1 million or 4 million infected Americans? How many of our teenagers can expect to be gravely ill in their 20's? We can better prepare for a deepening health care crisis and ensuing social upheaval.

Mandatory universal testing is a necessary component for preventing and controlling the AIDS epidemic. Prevention requires intervention. Intervention requires knowing who is positive. The alternative is today's catastrophic failure. Prevention is all we have. Education will only take us part of the way. The epidemic is proof of this. Anyone who preaches that education is our only hope for prevention must believe that there really is no hope!

The AIDS test is a laboratory measurement of HIV antibody. **The real test is how much we care about one another.**

ACROSS THE STREET FROM DISNEYLAND

35

It's a small world after all.

F rontierland. Fantasyland. Tomorrowland. We are like children lost in the park.

The California Medical Association (CMA) met at the Anaheim Convention Center, across from Disneyland, on March 6, 1995. By voice vote, 450 physician delegates requested that state legislation require anyone testing positive for HIV be reported to county health authorities. I applauded this first step. The vote was passed with wide recognition by the medical community that the AIDS epidemic is out of control and that there is desperate need of public health services to prevent transmission. The need to restore the principles of epidemiology was made clear, as was the need for early intervention.

Some characterized this vote as a sharp policy shift. It was an expression of concern by doctors, long overdue, but certainly welcome. These California physicians finally attempted to address AIDS as a communicable disease. They correctly pointed out the necessity of reporting everyone who tests HIV-positive in order to control the epidemic. But the vote clearly did *not* go far enough. *It did not call for mandatory testing to identify everyone infected.* What about the other 70% of people who are infected and have not been tested, and therefore, would not be reported? Adhering to the same social and medical concerns, it should be understood that this unidentified group is just as contagious and likely to spread this virus, leaving the same trail of suffering and death. It is necessary to identify and report everyone who is HIV-infected. *This requires that everyone be tested.*

Say it ain't so ... tell me it's not true! On March 5, 1996, one year later, CMA physician delegates again met across the street from Disneyland. They voted to rescind their own AIDS policy. Instead of supporting public health, they now chose to abandon public health. Instead of adopting a humane policy of mandatory testing, they abolished their earlier stand on mandatory reporting. One can only wonder why they didn't also vote to eliminate screening, reporting, and even treating other communicable diseases such as tuberculosis and gonorrhea. At the same time that these physicians were voting to do away with public health, their own children were visiting Disneyland. These are the children who now face a higher risk of dying of AIDS than of cancer or heart disease. Already one adolescent in this country becomes HIV-infected each hour. Our children will wander into Tomorrowland endangered by the cowardly decisions of their own parents (who are lost in Fantasyland).

Currently there are 22 to 30 million HIV casualties worldwide. The World Health Organization (WHO) now predicts there will be in excess of 40 million infected adults by the year 2000. The Harvard-based Global AIDS Policy Coalition (GAPC) has actually put this number as high as 110 million cases, including over 10 million infected children.

AIDS is exploding in India. Over half of Bombay's 100,000 women who work the brothels are already HIV-infected. Thousands of villages in Uganda are already decimated by AIDS. This Central African nation is estimated to have one million AIDS orphans by the year 1998. Thailand is predicted to have one million children and teens infected by the year 2000. The AIDS virus has also set its sites on the youth of

America—it's a small world after all.

In the summer of 1989, Jonathan Mann, then director of GAPC, while speaking at the Fifth International Conference on AIDS in Montreal, Canada, called for a new vision in approaching this pandemic. He properly criticized the lack of pragmatism. "To diffuse this global time bomb would require social adjustments, global solidarity, and a need to regard health as a central defining principle of local, national, and global purpose." He voiced how society and government needed to be held accountable for failed health policies.

Since the Montreal meeting there have been six more International AIDS Conferences held around the world. The news delivered at sessions in Yokohama, Japan, in 1994 was bad—no drug, no vaccine, no effective prevention. Total disappointment! It was decided to hold this meeting every other year instead of annually.

The 1996 AIDS conference concluded in Vancouver, Canada. It ushered in a new generation of expensive miracles. Many of those who attended the meeting were themselves HIV-infected and starved for hope. Research scientists in 1998 will try to explain the unfulfilled promises of Vancouver. The year 2000 might finally witness a *Declaration of Prevention!*

On March 10, 1995, a government release suggested that the severity of the AIDS epidemic was overstated. They reported that in the USA only 600,000 to 800,000 people were HIV-infected rather than 800,000 to 1.2 million. However, the reported number of full blown AIDS cases by December 1994 had exceeded 450,000 by our government's own statistics. Conservative estimates are that at least 3 times this number are HIV-infected, but in earlier stage disease, and not yet reported. Government policy allows no serious effort to find out true numbers. There has yet to be any official recommendation calling for universal screening.

The truth is no one knows the actual number of infections. We repeat each other's "guesstimates." All of the reported numbers are too high. These are death counts, not jelly beans in a jar. *Are we to thank the government for overestimating its original numbers, or to thank the virus for being six months behind schedule?*

Science cannot solve all human dilemmas. While we expect science to provide for our salvation, we forget science owes us no debt. We naively refuse to apply those epidemiologic tools that would allow us to better understand this disease and modify behavior.

AIDS has trashed epidemiology!

POINT OF NO RETURN

36

To die will be an awfully big adventure!
— Peter Pan (Sir J.M. Barrie)

A re we over the edge? When will it be too late even for intervention to halt this epidemic? Is it too late now? Many restless nights I have pondered these questions.

There is a trampling effect of HIV transmission. As more of the population becomes infected, the contagion pool increases. As the herd gets infected, any individual's chances of becoming newly infected increases. Only death, not cure, lowers the HIV saturation rate in the population. All interpersonal behavior becomes riskier as the infected population pool swells. Promiscuous behavior is more dangerous today than it has been at any other time. One might expect three random sexual exposures today to be as great a life-threatening risk as 25 random sexual exposures in 1981. The chance of coming in contact with contaminated blood at the scene of an auto accident is many times greater in 1996 than it was in 1985. This is because many more people are infected today. A seroprevalence study was conducted in Seattle, Washington, during the years 1989 to 1990 among adults treated for cardiac arrest before reaching a medical facility. The findings revealed that 0.8% of those people being resuscitated were HIV-positive. Does anyone wish to guess what this percentage will be by the year 2010?

The risk to health care workers from any accidental blood exposure progressively increases because more blood is contaminated. This risk will escalate daily as the epidemic gains momentum. All methods to control AIDS will become more difficult to implement as the percentage of the population which is HIV-positive increases. The financial resources available for each individual case and the manpower necessary to treat the larger number of cases will both be diminished proportionately.

If we've not yet slipped over the cliff, we are certainly pointed in that direction and moving ever so fast. There is an analogy of bacteria growing in a test tube of transparent broth culture media to help clarify this point. Try to imagine a certain bacteria that might multiply and double its population every thirty minutes. One bacteria becomes two. Two bacteria become four. Four bacteria become eight, and so on. For a period of time the contaminated broth media appears to be totally clear to the naked eye, and bacteria may even be difficult to see with a microscopic lens. Eventually a concentration of $5x10^4$ (50,000) bacteria per cubic millimeter of media is reached. The broth still appears clear to the naked eye. There are no apparent visual changes. Suddenly, thirty minutes later, the media turns cloudy. A critical threshold of 10^5 (100,000) bacteria per cubic millimeter has been attained. Even if there were a means to intervene at this point and immediately decrease the number of bacteria in half (back to $5x10^4$ concentration), again, in thirty minutes we would be right back to 10^5 bacteria, and once again the media would be clouded. If we could double the size of the container, in thirty minutes the broth would again reappear cloudy. We have reached a point of no return. With reference to the AIDS epidemic, I do not know if we are at $4x10^2$, $2x10^3$, or $8x10^4$.

Through the eyes of some, the AIDS broth has already begun to cloud.

WHERE THE RUBBER MEETS THE ROAD — *What I Tell My Children*

37

We are only one river. We are only one sea. And it flows through you, and it flows through me. We are only one people. We are one and the same. We are all one spirit. We are all one name. We are the father, mother, daughter and son. From the dawn of creation, we are one. We are one.

— *Peter Yarrow, "River of Jordan"*

I wish to share with the reader exactly how I present some important aspects of AIDS to my own children. I speak as a parent first, as a physician second.

I have three children. Their welfare is my responsibility. Jessica, Rhett, and Teague will be affected by AIDS throughout their lives. Their fate is woven into the fate of the world's children. Most people want the best for future generations. This will require controlling the AIDS epidemic. How much are we willing to sacrifice for this? Unchecked, AIDS will shortly be the world's leading cause of death. Each new case makes containment more difficult. AIDS will be responsible for unprecedented, terrifying social disintegration.

1. Daddy loves you. That never changes. It is difficult to be happy when you are sick. Happiness is the key to a good life. Stay healthy. People with AIDS are very ill. They would do anything to change their fate. They need help in living and in dying comfortably.

2. Everyone dies: you, me, mom, even those not yet born. The life cycle is bigger than any of

us. I hope your lives will be full. I hope they are filled with adventure and happiness. It is for you to create. Don't be afraid, just be careful.

3. You will hear a lot about AIDS statistics. Never forget that behind each number is a real person. Many of these people died too young, never allowed to reach life's full potential. Never forget "The Daedalus Project" AIDS benefit we shared together the summer of '95 in Ashland, Oregon. Never forget all the people who stood in memory of loved ones lost. Remember Ray Porter's song about the "museum of what could have been."

4. Your sexual preference is your own. It is not a decision; it is who you are. You are a human being first. Your creed, gender, and sexual preference are of lesser importance.

5. AIDS is not God's vengeance. It is an infectious disease caused by a virus. Social behavior is largely responsible for transmission. You are responsible for your social behavior. Sexual preference does not protect you from AIDS.

6. Not everything you hear about AIDS is true. Even what I tell you may not be correct in the future. Keep yourself informed.

7. The Golden Rule is for all time and all circumstances. Treat others as you would like them to treat you. Trust no religion or organization that is not consistent with this simple rule. This applies to AIDS—you do not want anyone to infect you with AIDS, you do not want to infect anyone else with AIDS.

8. Your health is precious. It's value is best measured when gone. AIDS is caused by a virus that will never leave your body. It always kills. There will be no cure in your lifetime. Unlike cancer or heart disease, it is spread from one person to another. Put in another way, everyone who is infected was infected by someone else. There is a chain of dying and suffering that you do not want to be part of.

9. If any of our family should ever acquire HIV, I expect we would all help each other through this tragedy. Your brothers and sisters extend beyond our immediate family. Remember this when you are older, even after Mom and Dad are gone.

10. Society is fast losing compassion. The human race is

being driven by money and greed. For HIV-infected people this turns a difficult life into a miserable existence. Be spiritually motivated in your life.

11. Don't be afraid to be tested for HIVirus. In the event you are infected, you must know it. Get early treatment and counseling. We, your parents, also want to know and be involved. No secret pinkie swears! If the entire world finds out, so be it. People who don't inform their family and friends often suffer the most. They also contribute to the stigma of this infection. Many gays have been conditioned to remain in the closet. The Gay Pride Parade in San Francisco demonstrates the relief of coming out and being oneself. If you are infected, this virus will someday show on your face. There is no spontaneous remission. Don't suffer alone in isolation.

12. One thing is worse than being infected with HIV—to infect someone else. The human suffering suddenly doubles. You will not survive, and now one more person will die unnecessarily. This virus does not differentiate first degree or second degree murder, manslaughter, or accident. The outcome is the same. Transmission is preventable. Your behavior must change if you become infected; your life becomes different. You are potentially very dangerous to others. Millions of people have died or are dying of AIDS because of the behavior of others. Lovers are killing lovers. Accept the fact your life has changed. Maintain your integrity. People will be more willing to assist you if they believe you would do nothing to harm them. Accept the fears of others at face value. They don't want what you have.

13. As long as you remain HIV-negative, never expose yourself to bodily secretions from someone who is HIV-positive or from a person whose HIV status you do not know. Make no exceptions. Even brushing your teeth creates abrasions that can allow this virus to enter your body. One mistake and your life is turned upside down. This epidemic is expanding! Any random exposure today carries a higher risk for HIV exposure than it did yesterday or anytime in the past. Ten thousand new people around the world become infected every day, each

one by someone else. Don't play Russian roulette, especially with more bullets than blanks.

14. If any of you children become HIV-infected keep your bodily secretions to yourself. They are never to be shared by anyone who is HIV-negative. Your blood is dangerous. Your saliva might be blood-contaminated. In my opinion, saliva by itself might be very dangerous. No French kissing or passionate kissing. Do not share razor blades, tooth brushes, or other instruments of hygiene. Be honest about your HIV status. Your status is someone else's business if you engage in any activity that endangers someone else's life.

15. Safe sex is no sex with anyone HIV-positive. Safe sex is no sex with anyone whose HIV status you do not know. The same goes for sharing saliva. Some proclaimed educators (who are not your parents) may disagree.

16. Unprotected sex with someone testing negative and whose background you are familiar with is safer than condom-protected sex with anyone whose HIV status is positive or not known. The failure rate of condoms resulting in pregnancy is 1 to 2% per month. Ten million infectious viral particles can fit through the same microscopic tear that a single sperm can squeeze through. Don't bet your life on a condom made of vinyl, latex, or steel. Always know the HIV status of your partner. If the status is unknown, even protected sex or sharing of saliva is a no-no. This virus gives you no second chance.

17. There is a vulnerable window period during which an HIV test may not yet indicate infectivity. This is the period of time it takes the body to develop detectable antibodies. Beware! A negative HIV antibody test is not a 100% guarantee of safety. Improved technology can shorten this window period from several months to several weeks. Antigen testing might further decrease this window period. As this epidemic progresses more HIV-infected people may be in this early window phase of disease. There is merit in the use of a condom for added protection. There is more merit in having this complemented with a negative antibody test and knowing the behavioral background of your partner.

18. If you ever become HIV-positive, you should only have sex or share secretions with someone who is also HIV-positive. Becoming infected with a second or multiple strains may present additional hazards. Indeed, most people with AIDS are probably already infected with multiple strains as a consequence of viral mutation and or repeated exposures. On balance, it is better to have one person infected with three strains of virus than three people infected with a single strain.

19. Life comes without a warranty. Do as I suggest and you can still get HIV-infected. An inadvertent needle stick, a blood splash, an unpredictable dental exposure, and rape are continuous risk factors. These risks increase as the epidemic intensifies. If you should be so unlucky, never hide your HIV status, never pass the virus to someone else...never pass the virus to someone else...never pass the virus to someone else...

20. By the way, while I'm at it, try cleaning your room sometime.

21. Daddy loves you. That never changes.

The End

ACKNOWLEDGMENTS

I have many people to thank. The best place to start is just next door. Ruth Orr turns 87 years young this year. She is the mother of the Peace Movement in Ventura County. She has organized four Great Books Clubs over the past 42 years. She still participates in all of them. Ruth has been a friend for 15 years and a next-door neighbor for 8 of those years. There are no fences between our homes or our hearts. She assisted me with each chapter, paragraph, word, and punctuation. She did not allow my pen to stray from my convictions. Pam and I love you very much.

Tim Robinson provided the "legs" for this book. I called upon his journalistic skills to help me put life into a story filled with human suffering and death. His insights made it easier for me to explain how humankind, by losing compassion for itself, can fuel an infectious epidemic. Tim, I can still hear your words, "Just say it like it is, just say it like it is." Thanks to you, I did.

Maurice Shimabuku. It wasn't fair how we became pals. I was asked to assist in the hospital care of your dying mother. She was too ill for me to have ever had the pleasure of knowing. Yet, she is the person responsible for acquainting us (Yin and Yang). We discovered that we lived just eleven doors apart. Our friendship continues to grow. You are the man: English teacher, motivator, coach. You are the incredible person that led the Port Hueneme Girls Volleyball Team to the California State Championship (and won). You assisted 36 young women to attain athletic scholarships. You gave my book the same attention you gave to your dying mother and to your dedicated students.

Gosta Iwasiuk, MD, provided valuable help in the writing of several chapters relating to the risk of AIDS to health care workers. He shared his perspective as a practicing surgeon and his concerns as a father and husband. His contribution included his wife, Mary Iwasiuk. Mary made this project so much easier. Between her animals, lemons, and avocados, she was still able to leave enough room for me. When I asked for her help in editing, I had no idea she would so skillfully unravel many of my thoughts into the right words.

Peng Fan, MD, was one of the first physicians to describe the AIDS syndrome in early 1981. Many, including myself, regard Peng as one of America's brightest physicians. I first became acquainted with Peng in 1973 when I was fortunate to serve as an intern under his tutelage as a medical resident. He taught me how to place chest tubes and aspirate bone marrows. He also introduced me to chow fun noodles. He taught me that practicing medicine is a privilege. Peng has been a friend ever since. I am grateful for his insightful suggestions regarding the manuscript.

I am forever indebted to Charles and Sylvia Savitch who played a major role in emotionally supporting me throughout the writing of this book. Early on, they provided me with the tools to obtain an education and follow a career in medicine. My parents, along with my grandparents, Becky and Jake Yudson, remain my best teachers of tolerance and love.

Jessica Savitch, you typed and retyped. This is how you spent your entire spring break from school—you raised the curtain for *Nutcracker.* These were the core chapters from which I was able to create a book. How does one thank a child for such devotion? I hope I have many seasons to figure that out.

Victoria Givens and I have worked together for eleven years. I am certain that all of our patients appreciated her warmth and kindness. Many of these people were dying of AIDS. She made their lives more comfortable and my job that much easier.

There was a bull in Mexico, slaughtered 45 years ago, to whom I must pay homage. Marcelo Gonzalez was a young ranch hand in Aqua Caliente, Mexico. In 1944 he was gored by a bull that left him with a chronic infection of the femur. When this infection flared up in 1989 his 17 year-old daughter, Margie, brought him to my office. I was not only impressed with the story behind his infection, but I was moved by the patience and respect Margie showed her father. A short while later Margie Gonzalez came to work for me. The attention she gives to her father is the same that she gives to all of our patients. This is an exceptional quality in the midst of health care delivery becoming more impersonal. Margie entered nursing school this past year. She already is ahead of the task; she understands the most important part of patient care.

A special thanks to Henry Oster, MD, whom I have worked closely with for the past 16 years. We have shared in the care of many patients. Together we have watched this epidemic take too many people.

Randy Shilts provided inspiration. He covered the AIDS epidemic for the *San Francisco Chronicle.* He monitored the beat of the epidemic, the beat of our species. I first read his book while on a holiday in Nova Scotia in 1988. Perhaps it was no coincidence that I finished the last chapter of his book while perched on a rock next to a lighthouse. The warning that day was clear. His culminating story, *And the Band Played On,* is the epitaph of public health failure. In Shilts' own words, "The bitter truth is that AIDS did not just happen to America— it was allowed to happen by an array of institutions, all of which failed to perform their appropriate tasks to safeguard the public health." I hope my story can stand as a small lighthouse next to the larger one Randy Shilts left us. Randy Shilts died of AIDS on February 12, 1994. His message should live in our hearts and guide our actions.

In October of 1978, while working in the emergency room at a University of California Hospital, I was the recipient of the projectile vomitus of a young overdose patient. It was 3:00 a.m. I wasn't alone. A nursing student whom I had never met before was also splashed. We cleaned ourselves up and then got married. We now have three children. Pam co-authored this book but refuses to take credit (or blame). She treated each revision of the manuscript as though it was a sick child. Many of the phrases are hers. Apologies to Pam's tennis partners for my frequently stealing her away.

My gratitude is extended to James Herman, MD, and Gretchen Jacobson, MD, neurosurgeons *par excellence.* Their skill in mending my health allowed me to continue my work on this book.

Others who have reviewed the manuscript and offered useful suggestions include: Nancy Mitchell RN, Melvin Cheatham MD, Cheryll Smith PhD, Carol Milligan MD, Angela Rabkin MD, Fred Payne MD, Bud Sloan DVM, Gordon Johnston MD, Larry Kozek DDS, Celia Hartley RN, Bill Eastman, Shepherd Smith, Roshan Shah MD, Charles Hollingsworth MD, Assibi Abudu MD, Nettie Mayersohn, Charles Rabkin MD, and Ralph Frerichs PhD, DVM.

For technical support I would also like to thank: Annie and Don Bates, Joanne Kennedy, Shelley Kozek, Joel and Kay Newsom, Frances Schnabel, Jorge and Cheryl Maradiegue, David Golden, Garren Mizutani, Wendy Miller, Linda Doyle RN, Carolyn Shimabuku, Maria Jimenez, Linda Hardison, Robert Rabkin MD, Bud Wakefield, Ari Bloom, Tom and Karen Pecht, Loise Ordner, John O'Brien PharmD, Eugene Fussell MD, Phyllis Amerikaner, Kooros Parsa MD, Leigh Gori, Richard Smith, Scott Voorman MD, John Orr, Ann Chung, Michelle Arya RN, Joe Morales, Joe Urango RN, Elizabeth Bergman RN, Judy McDonald RN, Dana and Janet Eaton, Sandra Lang RN, Joyce Jones, Martin and April Riessen, Mack

McCurdy, Hans Wortelkamp, Rob Bagdazian, Albert Amorteguy MD, Ann Hansen, Thomas Kong MD, Christine O'Neill, David Wood, Janice Birlenbach, Marge Prince RN, Patty Paumier, Susan Becker RN, Francine Sewall, Mary Jo Garrett RN, and Sandra Smith.

Thank you to Eleanor Sandstrom, Gayle Engle, Roland Gardner, Sue Johnston, Eva Ettedgui RN, Howard Sandler, and Kimberley Cameron for your undying enthusiasm.

Many of my patients and their surviving friends and family have given me emotional support. Most of these people are not specifically mentioned in this book. Witnessing their heroic battles in the face of personal tragedy inspired me to offer my version of this medical calamity. The story that resulted is not uplifting, but I hope it will convince us that it will take *more than* marches, galas, and fund-a-thons to prevent the HIVirus from infecting more people. Unless public health is resurrected and human compassion restored countless more will die in the AIDS epidemic—some to be remembered as a patch on a quilt, others to be forgotten in unmarked graves.

Nick Baiamonte is one patient to whom I owe a particular debt of gratitude. He became a close friend. He was always scheduled late afternoons because of his job commitments. Nick became especially well acquainted with my office staff. We talked about everything from politics to what it was once like to feel healthy and happy. Nick, I still have two of the bottles of ale you entered in the State Fair. I use them as book ends. They remind me of our friendship. I drank the third. You offered many useful suggestions for this book which I now share with others. I miss you.

To Jessica, Rhett, and Teague Savitch—you are why this book was written.

ABOUT THE AUTHOR

D r. Cary Savitch received his medical degree from the University of California, San Francisco. He is board certified in Internal Medicine and Infectious Diseases. In 1980 he completed a Fellowship in Infectious Diseases at the University of California, San Francisco.

Dr. Savitch is presently a Fellow of the American College of Physicians. He has been an Assistant Clinical Professor of Medicine at UCLA for the past 15 years. He is in private medical practice on the central coast of California where he lives with his wife and three children. He is a past president of the Ventura County Chapter of Physicians for Social Responsibility and has also been a member of the International Physicians for the Prevention of Nuclear War. He is co-founder of HEALR (Health Educators Advocating Legal Reform), and has served on various AIDS Task Forces. He lectures on AIDS and other topics relating to Infectious Diseases.

REFERENCES

The following references selected by the author were found to be most applicable to the chapters listed. These articles and texts were selected to provide a balanced point of view. The conclusions drawn in many of the articles are not necessarily shared by the author. Most of the statistics used in this book are sourced from the references below or obtained from material furnished at Infectious Disease conferences. Because the practice of public health is so compromised many statistics lack the verification satisfactory to the author.

2. ICE AIDS: IN THE END

2-1. Gore R. Extinctions- What Caused Earth's Great Dyings? *National Geographic.* Jun 1989;175(6):662-699.

2-2. Myers, G. HIV: Its origin and its future. *HIV, Advances in Research and Therapy.* Oct 1993;3:3-10.

5. ONE STRIKE AND YOU'RE OUT

5-1. Cote TR, et al. Risk of suicide among persons with AIDS. *JAMA* 1992;268(15):2066-2068.

5-2. Battin MP. Physicians, partners, and people with AIDS: deciding about suicide. *Crisis.* 1994;15(1):15-21, 43.

5-3. Breitbart W, et al. Interest in physician-assisted suicide among ambulatory HIV-infected patients. *Am J Psychiatry.* Feb,1996;153(2):238-242.

5-4. Winker MA, et al. Infectious diseases. A global approach to a global problem. *JAMA.* Jan 17, 1996;275(3):245-246.

5-6. Gromyko A, et al. *Breakthrough.* Walker and Company, New York. 1988.

6. THE OAKLAND AIDS BRIDGE MEETS THE GOLDEN GAY BRIDGE

6-1. Sande MA, et al. _The Medical Management of AIDS._ Philadelphia: W.B. Saunders Co, 1994, 90-91.

6-2. Gilden D. The Saint of Castro Street. _PAACNOTES._ 1992;4(5):252-255.

6-3. Laurence J. AIDS: The second decade. _Infections in Med supplement._ Oct 1992;9(F):4-5.

6-4. Heterosexually acquired AIDS-United States, 1993. _MMWR._ Mar 11, 1994;43(9):155-160.

6-5. Jaret P. Viruses. _National Geographic._ July 1994;186(1):58-91.

6-6. Hagn B. Origin and evolution of primate lentiviruses. _AIDS Reader Supplement._ Nov/Dec 1995:16-17.

7. YOUR DOC CAN'T SAVE YOU

7-1. Vermund SH, et al. Epidemiology and public health impact of HIV infection and AIDS. _Comprehensive management of HIV Disease: HIV Speakers' Forum 1V Annual Update Meeting_ Nov 18-21 1993, Phoenix, Arizona, Summary Report pg 5.

7-2. State of California - Health and Welfare Agency. HIV-Related Mortality Trends Among Adults Aged 25 to 44 years in California, 1987-1993. _California Morbidity._ March 10, 1995 (no. 9, no. 10).

7-3. Selik RM, et al. HIV infection as the leading cause of death among young adults in US cities and states. _JAMA._ 1993;269:2991-2994.

7-4. Update: AIDS among women - United States, 1994. _MMWR._ 1995;44(5):81-84.

7-5. Bryson YJ, et al. Clearance of HIV infection in a perinatally infected infant. _N Engl J Med._ 1995;332:833-838.

7-6. Rudin C, et al. Transient infection in human immunodeficiency virus type 1- exposed infants. _Ped Infec Dis J._ Feb, 1996;15(2):182.

7-7. Bakshi SS, et al. Repeatedly positive human immunodeficiency virus type 1 DNA polymerase chain reaction in human immunodeficiency virus-exposed seroreverting infants. _Pediatr Infect Dis J._ 1995;14:658-662.

7-8. Klein RS, et al. Transmission of human immunodeficiency virus type 1 (HIV-1) by exposure to blood: defining the risk. _Ann Intern Med._ Nov 15, 1990;113(10):729-730.

7-9. Donegan E, et al. Infection with human immunodeficiency virus type 1 (HIV-1) among recipients of antibody-positive blood donations. _Ann of Intern Med._ 1990;113:733-739.

7-10. Cao YU, et al. Virologic and immunologic characterization of long-term survivors of human immunodeficiency virus type 1 infection. _N Engl J Med._ 1995;332:201-208.

7-11. Pantaleo G, et al. Studies in subjects with long-term nonprogressive human immunodeficiency virus infection. _N Engl J Med._ 1995;332(4):209-216.

7-12. Baltimore D. Lessons from People with Nonprogressive HIV Infection. _N Eng J Med._ 1995; 332(4):259-260.

7-13. Baker, B. Long-term HIV survivors hold treatment clues. _Internal Med News._ Sept 15, 1995;28(18):36.

7-14. Levy JA. Long-term survivors of HIV infection. _Hospital Prac._ Oct 15, 1994:41-52.

7-15. Huanag Y, et al. Characterization of nef Sequences in Long-Term Survivors of Human Immunodeficiency Virus Type 1 Infection. *J Virology.* 1995, Jan;69(1):93-100.

7-16. Learmont J, et al. Long-term symptomless HIV-1 infection in recipients of blood products from a single donor. *Lancet.* Oct 1992;340(8824):863-867.

7-17. Haynes WS, et al. Factors influencing long-term nonprogression of HIV disease. *The AIDS Reader.* Dec 1994;4(6):199-203.

7-18. Ho DD. Plenary Session: Long-Term Nonprogressors (abstract PS10). *The AIDS Reader Supplement. Tenth International Conference on AIDS, Yokohama,* Aug 7-12, 1994:3.

7-19. Two reports from Asia show rapid HIV spread. *PAACNOTES.* Aug 1993:354.

7-20. The time is running out in Asia. *AIDS Today - highlights from the tenth international conference on AIDS.* Aug 8-12, 1994:3-5. Yokohama, Japan.

7-21. Celentano DD, et al. Risk factors for HIV-1 seroconversion among young men in Northern Thailand. *JAMA.* Jan 10, 1996;275(2):122-127.

7-22. Chaisson RE. HIV infection: The world picture in 1992. *Infections in Med Supplement.* Oct 1992;9(F):6-10.

7-23. Pinner, RW, et al. Trends in infectious diseases mortality in the United States. *JAMA.* Jan 17, 1996;275(3):189-193.

7-24. World Population Profile: 1994, May: U.S. Department of Commerce.

8.   THE OTHER CASTRO

8-1. Wald K, et al. Viva las Vegas? Cuba's AIDS policy earns some surprising support. *Frontiers.* Jun 17, 1994:15-18.

8-2. de Gordon AM, et al. Cuban AIDS policy. *Lancet.* Dec 4, 1993; 342(8884):1426.

8-3. Moas C, et al. AIDS policy and HIV epidemic in Cuba. *Int Conf AIDS.* 1990 Jun 20-23;6(2):105 (abstract no. F.D.64).

8-4. Scheper-Hughes N. AIDS, public health, and human rights in Cuba. *Lancet.* Oct 16, 1993;342:965-967.

9.   TODAY

9-1. Notification of syringe-sharing and sex partners of HIV-infected persons - Pennsylvania, 1993-1994. *MMWR.* Mar 24, 1995;44(11):202-204.

10.   WALT WENT NUTS!

10-1. Portegies, P. AIDS Dementia Complex: A Review. *Journal of Acquired Immune Deficiency Syndromes.* 7(Supp. 2) 1994:S38-S49.

10-2. Koppel BS. New developments in the pathophysiology and treatment of the AIDS dementia complex. *The AIDS Reader.* Jan/Feb 1995:6-12.

10-3 Price RW, et al. The brain in AIDS; central nervous system HIV-1 infection and AIDS dementia complex. *Science.* 1988; 239:586-592.

12.   ALL THE SURVIVORS ARE DEAD

12-1. Laurence J. The frustrating challenge of HIV therapeutics. *AIDS Reader.* Sept/Oct 1995;5(5):147-150.

12-2. Fischl MA, et al. The efficacy of azidothymidine (AZT) in the treatment of patients with AIDS and AIDS-related complex: A double-blind, placebo-controlled trial. *N Engl J Med.* 1987;317:185-191.

12-3.   Fischl MA, et al. The safety and efficacy of zidovudine (AZT) in the treatment of subjects with mildly symptomatic human immunodeficiency virus type 1 (HIV) infection: A double-blind, placebo-controlled trial. *Ann Intern Med.* 1990;112:727-737.

12-4.   Volberding PA, et al: Zidovudine in asymptomatic human immunodificiency virus infection. *N Engl J Med.* Apr 5, 1990;322:941-949.

12-5.   Kuritzkes D. Impact of therapy on survival in HIV infection. *HIV/AIDS Clinical Insight.* Nov 1992;3(1):2-5.

12-6.   Mascolini, M. Outsiders and insiders explore ins and outs of HIV clinical trials. *J Phys Asso AIDS Care.* May 1994;5:11-16.

12-7.   Hamilton JD, et al. A controlled trial of early versus late treatment with zidovudine in symptomatic human immunodeficiency virus infection. *N Engl Med.* 1992;326:437-443.

12-8.   Concord Coordinating Committee. Concorde: MRC/ANRS randomised double-blind controlled trial of immediate deferred zidovudine in symptom-free HIV infection. *Lancet.* 1994;343:871-881.

12-9   Aboulker JP, et al. Preliminary analysis of the Concorde trial. *Lancet.* 1993;341:889-890.

12-10. AZT and Survival, Concords results. *Lancet.* Apr 9, 1994;343:866-867.

12-11. Diminishing Returns: Another European study. *JAMA.* Apr 13,1994; 271:1088-1092.

12-12. Fischl MA, et al. Combination and monotherapy with zidovudine and zalcitabine in patients with advanced HIV disease. The NIAID AIDS Clinical Trials Group. *Annals of Internal Med.* Jan 1, 1995;122(1):24-32.

12-13. Rabkin JG. Conversations with AIDS Specialists. *PAACNOTES.* 1993;5(4):128-132.

12-14. Cassens B. Drug interactions in the treatment of HIV disease. *Clinical Insight.* April 1993;3(3):4-7.

12-15. Antiretroviral Resistance. *International AIDS Society-USA.* Aug 1994;2(2):6-8.

12-16. Schooley RT. Fifth European conference on clinical aspects and treatment of AIDS. *HIV Information Network.* FAX newsletter (sponored by Univ Alabama Sch Med) Oct 12, 1995.

12-17. Fogelman I, et al. Prevalence and patterns of use of concomitant medications among participants in three multicenter HIV type 1 clinical trials. *J AIDS.* 1994;7:1057-1063.

12-18. New NIH AIDS policy decrees more laboratory-initiated research. *Internal Medicine World Report.* Mar 1995;10(6):13.

12-19. AIDS 1994: A time capsule of the year's events. *Int Med World Report.* Nov 1-14 1994;9(19):10-14.

12-20. Senterfill W. A new twist on early AZT use. *Being Alive. People with HIV/ AIDS Action Coalition Newsletter.* April 1994:1.

12-21. ZDV monotherapy has no detectable anti-HIV effect in early HIV disease. *Infectious Disease News.* May 1996;9(5):22.

12-22. Lenderking WR, et al. Evaluation of the quality of life associated with zidovudine treatment in asymptomatic human immunodeficiency virus infection. *New Engl J Med.* March 17, 1994;330(11):738-743.

12-23. Fauci A. New Drugs in the War on AIDS. *U.S. News and World Report.* Dec 25, 1995;119(25):80.

12-24. Danner SA, et al. A short-term study of the safety, pharmacokinetics, and efficacy of ritonavir, an inhibitor of HIV-1 protease. *N Engl J Med.* Dec 7, 1995;333(23):1528-1533.

12-25. Markowitz M, et al. A preliminary study of ritonavir, an inhibitor of HIV-1 protease, to treat HIV-1 infection. *N Engl J Med.* Dec 7, 1995;333(23):1534-1539.

12-26. Montaner JSG, et al. Combination therapy for the treatment of HIV disease: Overcoming HIV drug resistance. *AIDS Reader Supplement.* Nov/ Dec 1995:5.

12-27. Mellors JW, et al. Quantitation of HIV-1 RNA in plasma predicts outcome after seroconversion. *Ann Intern Med.* 1995;122:573-579.

12-28. Carey, J. AIDS: Maybe there isn't a magic bullet. *Business Week.* Oct. 24, 1994:108-109.

12-29. Healea, T. Three Hits, No Home Run. *POZ.* Feb/Mar. 1996;(12):19.

13.   VACCINE PROOF?

13-1.   Rowland-Jones S, et al. HIV-specific cytotoxic T-cells in HIV-exposed but uninfected Gambian women. *Nat Med.* 1995;1(1):59-64.

13-2.   Carmichael A, et al. *Medicine a Treasury of Art and Literature.* Hugh Lauter Levin Assoc, Inc., New York. 1991.

13-3   Samson M, et al. Resistance to HIV-1 infection in caucasian individuals bearing mutant alleles of the CCR-5 chemokine receptor gene. *Nature* Aug 1996;382:722-725.

13-4.   Chang NT. The search for an AIDS vaccine. *AIDS Reader.* 1994;4(2):45-49.

13-5.   HIV Vaccine; Dilemmas in development. *AIDS Today - highlights from the tenth international conference on AIDS.* Aug 8-12, 1994:10-11. Yokohama, Japan.

13-6.   Caldwell M. The Long Shot. *Discover.* Aug,1993:61-70.

13-7.   Charnow JA. Expanded HIV vaccine trials put on hold. Infectious *Disease News.* Aug 1994;7(8):1,20.

13-8.   Oliwenstein L. AIDS-1992, Modeling the Plague. *Discover.* Jan 1993;14 (1):64.

13-9.   Hu DJ, et al. The emerging genetic diversity of HIV. *JAMA.* Jan 17, 1996;275(3):210-216.

13-10. O'Brien WA, et al. Changes in plasma HIV-1 RNA and CD4+ lymphocyte counts and the risk of progression to AIDS. *N Engl J Med.* Feb 15, 1996;334 (7):426-431.

13-11. Update on the Baboon-marrow transplant. *HIV Hotline.* Jan/Feb 1996;6(1):7.

13-12. Jackson GG, et al. Passive immunoneutralization of human immunodeficiency virus in patients with advanced AIDS. *Lancet.* 1988;2:647-652.

15.   EARLY INTERVENTION
For Treatment And Prevention

15-1.   Ho DD, et al. Rapid turnover of plasma virions and CD4 lymphocytes in HIV-1 infection. *Nature.* 1995;373(12):123-126.

15-2.   Connor EM et al. Reduction of maternal-infant transmission of human immunodificiency virus type 1 with zidovudine treatment. *N Engl J Med.* Nov 3,1994;331:1173-1180.

15-3.   Zidovudine for the prevention of HIV transmission from mother to infant. *MMWR.* April 29, 1994;43(16):285-287.

15-4.   Wilfert, CM. Just Do It. Interrupting maternal-to-infant transmission of HIV. *HIV Newsline.* Oct 1995:1(5):77-81.

15-5.   Dickover RE, et al. Identification of levels of maternal HIV-1 RNA asociated with risk of perinatal transmission. *JAMA.* Feb 28, 1996; 275(8):599-605.

15-6.   Prazuck T, et al. Mother-to-child transmission of human immunideficiency virus type 1 and type 2 and dual infection: a cohort study in Banfora, Burkina Faso. *Pediatric Infec Dis J.* Nov 1995; 14(11):940-947.

15-7.   Recommendations of the US public health service task force on the use of Zidovudine to reduce perinatal transmission of human immunodeficiency virus. *MMWR.* 1994;43(No RR-11):1-20.

15-8.   Fleischman AR, et al. Mandatory Newborn Screening for HIV. *AIDS Reader.* 1994, Sept/Oct:172-175.

15-9.   Davis SF, et al. Prevalence and incidence of vertically acquired HIV infection in the United States. *JAMA.* 1995;274(12):952-955.

15-10.   Golden DA. The effects of testing and behavior change on dynamic modeling of HIV/AIDS. May 1, 1995. A Senior Thesis presented to the Faculty of the Woodrow Wilson School of Public and International Affairs, Princeton University.

15-11.   Archer VE. Psychological defenses and control of AIDS. *Am J Public Health.* 1989;79:876-878.

15-12.   Higgens, DL, Evidence for the effects of HIV antibody counseling and testing on risk behaviors, *JAMA.* Nov 6, 1991,266(17):2419-29.

15-13.   Wenger NS. Reduction of high-risk sexual behavior among heterosexuals undergoing HIV antibody testing: a randomized clinical trial. *Amer J Pub Health.* Dec 1991;81(12):1580-1586.

15-14.   Cleary PD. Behavior changes after notification of HIV infection. *Amer J Pub Health.* Dec 1991;81(12):1586-1591.

15-15.   van Griensven GJ, et al. Effect of human immunodeficiency virus (HIV) antibody knowledge on high-risk sexual behavior with steady and nonsteady sexual partners among homosexual men. *Am J Epidemiol.* 1989;129:596-603.

15-16.   Higgins DL, et al. Evidence for the effects of HIV antibody counseling and testing on risk behaviors. *JAMA.* 1991;266:2419-2429.

15-17.   Makadon HJ, et al. Prevention of HIV infection in primary care: current practices, future possibilities. *Ann Intern Med.* 1995;123:715-719.

15-18.   Selected behaviors that increase risk for HIV infection, other sexually transmitted diseases, and unintended pregnancy among high school students - United States, 1991. *MMWR.* 1992:41(50):945-950.

15-19.   HIV Counseling and testing- United States, 1993. *MMWR.* 1995;44(9):169-174.

15-20.   Hinman AR. Strategies to prevent HIV infection in the United States. *Am J Public Health.* 1991;81:1557-1559.

15-21.   Chaisson RE, et al. Pneumocystis prophylaxis and survival in patients with advanced human immunodeficiency virus infection treated with zidovudine. *Arch Intern Med.* 1992;152:2009-2013.

15-22.   Ioannidis JP, et al. Early or deferred zidovudine therapy in HIV-infected patients without an AIDS-defining illness. *Ann Intern Med.* 1995;122:856-866.

15-23. Mascolini, M. Europeans' defiant optimism demands early intervention, individualized care. *J Physicians Assoc for AIDS Care.* Apr 1994;1:6-14.

15-24. U.S. public health service recommendations for human immunodeficiency virus counseling and voluntary testing for pregnant women. *MMWR.* July 1995;44(No. RR-7):1-15.

15-25. AIDS will orphan more than 80,000 children by the year 2000. *PAACNOTES.* Dec 1992:409.

17. HEADS IN CEMENT

17-1. Fiore F. White House AIDS activist falls into political exile. *Los Angeles Times.* Sept 11, 1995:A1.

17-2. Des Jarlais DC, et al. Antibodies to a retrovirus etiologically associated with acquired immunodeficiency syndrome in populations with increased incidence of the syndrome. *MMWR.* July 13, 1984;33(27):377-379.

17-3. Barre-Sinoussi F, et al. Isolation of a T-lymphotropic retrovirus from a patient at risk for acquired immune deficiency syndrome (AIDS). *Science.* 1983;220:868-871.

17-4. Gallo RC, et al. Frequent detection and isolation of cytopathic retroviruses (HTLV-III) from patients with AIDS and at risk for AIDS. *Science.* 1984;224:500-503.

17-5. Addressing emerging infectious disease threats: A prevention strategy for the United States Executive Summary. *MMWR.* Apr 15, 1994;43(RR-5):1-18.

17-6. Ward JW, et al. Recommendations for HIV testing services for inpatients and outpatients in acute-care hospital settings. *MMWR.* Jan 15, 1993;42:1-6.

18. IRON CURTAIN DOWN: AIDS CURTAIN UP

18-1. Decree of the Presidium of the Supreme Soviet of the USSR on measures to prevent infection with the AIDS virus. *J Med Philos.* 1989 Jun;14(3):359-360.

18-2. Lange WR. HIV screening of travelers to eastern Europe. *Postgrad Med.* 1991 Sept 15;90(4):26.

20. EDUCATE THE EDUCATORS

20-1. Elias C, Nonoxynol-9: The Need for Policy in the Face of Uncertainty. *AIDS.* 1995;9(3):311-312.

20-2. Weller SC. Meta-Analysis of Condom Effectiveness in Reducing Sexually Transmitted HIV. *Soc Sci Med.* 1993; 36(12):1735-1744.

20-3. Update: Barrier protection against HIV infection and other sexually transmitted diseases. *MMWR.* Aug 6, 1993;42(30):589-591.

20-4. Voeller B, et al. Mineral Oil Lubricants Cause Rapid Deterioration of Latex Condoms. *Contraception.* 1989; 39(1):95-101.

20-5. Kreiss J, et al. Efficacy of Nonoxynol 9 contraceptive sponge use in preventing heterosexual acquisition of HIV in Nairobi postitutes. *JAMA.* 1992;268(4):477-482.

20-6. Boxall B. Young Gays Stray From Safe Sex, New Data Shows. *Los Angeles Times.* Sept 3, 1995:A1,24.

20-7. HIV spreading among young men despite warning, study shows. *HIV Hotline.* Jan/Feb, 1996;6(1):9.

20-8.   Spayde J, et al. 100 visionaries who could change your life. *UTNE Reader.* Jan-Feb 1995;67:54-81.

20-9.   Aita, K.. HIV hemophiliacs vow to continue fight for apology. *The Japan Times.* Oct 16-22, 1995:4.

20-10. MacGregor HE. Japan official apologizes in AIDS scandal. *Los Angeles Times.* Feb 17, 1996:A1,A7.

20-11. Editors. The shift in trends of HIV infection, A global picture. *The AIDS Reader.* Mar/Apr1993;3(2)37-39.

20-12. Selected behaviors that increase risk for HIV infection among high school students - United States, 1990. *MMWR.* Apr 10, 1992;41(14):231-240.

20-13. HIV still on the rise among teens. *Infectious Disease News.* Jan 1996;9(1):1.

20-14. Ronge LJ. Slowing the spread of HIV among teens requires awareness, education. *Infectious Disease News.* Jan 1996;9(1):6.

20-15. Seroconversion to simian immunodeficiency virus in two lab workers. *MMWR.* 1992;41:678-681.

20-16. Wahn V, et al. Horizontal transmission of HIV infection between two siblings. *Lancet.* Sept 20, 1986;2:694.

20-17. HIV transmission between two adolescent brothers with hemophilia. *MMWR.* Dec.17,1993;42(49):948-951.

20-18. HIV infection in two brothers receiving intravenous therapy for hemophilia. *MMWR.* Apr 10, 1992;42(14):228-231.

20-19. Apparent transmission of human T-lymphocyte virus type III/ lymphadenopathy-associated virus from a child to a mother providing health care. *MMWR.* 1986;35:76-79.

20-20. Human Immunodeficiency virus transmission in household settings-United States. *MMWR.* 1994;43(19):347-356.

20-21. Fitzgibbon, et al. Transmission from one child to another of human immunodeficiency virus type 1 with a zidovudine-resistance mutation. *N Engl J Med.* 1993;329 (25):1835-1841.

20-22. Shirley LR et al. Risk of transmission of human immunodeficiency virus by bite of an infected toddler. *J Pediatr.* 1989;114:425-427.

20-23. Richman KM, et al. The potential for transmission of human immunodeficiency virus through human bites. *J Acquired Imm Def Synd.* 1993;6:402-406.

20-24. Rozsa L, et al. Prostitute's bite transmits AIDS virus. *The Herald (Miami).* Oct 27, 1995.

20-25. Anonymous. Transmission of HIV by human bite. Lancet 1987;2:522.

20-26. Dushaiko GM, et al. Hepatitis C virus transmitted by human bite. *Lancet.* 1990;336:504.

20-27. Hamilton JD et al. Transmission of hepatitis B by a human bite; an occupational hazard. *Can Med Assoc J.* 1976;115:439-440.

20-28. MacQuarrie MB et al. Hepatitis B transmitted by a human bite. *JAMA.* 1974;230:723-724.

20-29. Cancio-Bello TP et al. An institutional outbreak of hepatitis B related to a human biting carrier. *J Infect Dis.* 1982;146:652-656.

20-30. Piazza M, et al. Passionate kissing and microlesions of the oral mucosa: Possible role in AIDS transmission. *JAMA.* Jan 13, 1989;261(2):244-245.

20-31. Woolley RJ. The biologic possibility of HIV transmission during passionate kissing. *JAMA.* 1989;262:2230.

20-32. Levy JA et al. HIV in saliva. *Lancet.* 1988;2:1248.

20-33. Groopman JE et al. HTLV-III in saliva of people with AIDS-related complex and healthy homosexual men at risk for AIDS. *Science.* 1984;226:447-449.

20-34. Barr CE, et al. Recovery of infectious HIV-I from whole saliva. *J Am Dent Assoc.* 1992;123:37-45.

20-35. Fox PC. Salivary gland involvement in HIV-1 infection. *Oral Surg Oral Med Oral Pathol.* 1992 Feb;73 (2):168-170.

20-36. Fox PC et al. Salivary inhibition of HIV-I infectivity; functional properties and distribution in men, women, and children. *J Am Dent Assoc.* 1989;118:709-711.

20-37. Yolken RH, et al. Persistent diarrhea and fecal shedding of retroviral nucleic acids in children infected with human immunodeficiency virus. *J Infec Dis.* 1991;164:61-66.

20-38. Supapannachart N, et al. Isolation of human immunodeficiency virus type 1 in cutaneous blister fluid. *Arch Dermatol.* 1991;127:1198-1200.

20-39. HIV infection and AIDS-A status report. *Surgeon General's Report to the American Public on HIV Infection and AIDS.* Printed by National Institutes of Health, June 1993:1,8.

20-40. California Department of Health Services Office of AIDS. Oral Sex: Recommendations from the California Department of Health Services, Office of AIDS. *HIV Education and Prevention Services Bulletin.* Oct/Nov 1993;1.

20-41. Department of Health Services, Office of AIDS. How to reduce risk of HIV infection during oral sex. *HIV Education and Prevention Services Bulletin.* Dec/Jan 1994.

20-42. Rozenbaum W, et al. HIV transmission by oral sex. *Lancet.* Jun 18, 1988:1395.

20-43. Laurence J. The Risk of HIV transmission from oral-genital intercourse. *The AIDS Reader.* Aug 1994;4(4):123-124.

20-44. Seibt AC, et al. Condom use and sexual identity among men who have sex with men-Dallas, 1991. *MMWR.* Jan 15, 1993;42(1):7-13.

20-45. Frank T. Relapse: Don't Do It. Advice from an AIDS educator who knows. *POZ.* Oct 1995;10:26,61.

20-46. Curran JW, et al. Epidemiology of HIV infection and AIDS in the United States. *Science.* Feb 5, 1988;239:610-616.

20-47. AIDS risk behaviors high among Americans older than age 50. *Internal Medicine World Report.* Aug 1994:16,33.

20-48. Cohen J. SIV data raise concern on oral-sex risk. *Science.* Jun 7, 1996; 272:1421-1422.

20-49. Baba TW, et al. Infection and AIDS in adult macaques after nontraumatic oral exposure to cell-free SIV. *Science.* Jun 7, 1996;272:1486-1489.

22. YOUR WORST TOOTHACHE

22-1. Lifson AR. Do alternate modes for transmission of human immunodeficiency virus exist? *JAMA.* 1988 Mar 4;259(9):1353-1356.

22-2. Gilbert DN. Patients with Human Immunodeficiency Virus Infection in the Hemodialysis Unit. *Arch Intern Med.* 1995;155:1576.

22-3. Serb P, et al. HIV infection and the dentist: The presence of HIV in saliva and its implications to dental practice. *Aust Dent J.* 1994 Apr;39(2):67-72.

22-4.   Gerbert B, et al. Possible health care professional-to-patient HIV transmission: dentists' reactions to a centers for disease control report. *JAMA.* 1991;265:1845-1848.

22-5.   Blank S, et al. Possible nosocomial transmission of HIV. *Lancet.* 1994;344:512-514.

22-6.   HIV instruction and selected HIV-risk behaviors among high school students-United States, 1989-1991. *MMWR.* Nov 20, 1992;41(46):866-868.

22-7.   Chant K, et al. Patient-to patient transmission of HIV in private surgical consulting rooms. *Lancet.* Dec 18,1993;342:Letters to the Editor.

22-8.   Possible transmission of human immunodeficiency virus to a patient during an invasive dental procedure. *MMWR.* July 27,1990;39(29):489-492.

22-9.   Ciesielski C, et al. Transmission of human immunodeficiency virus in a dental practice. *Ann Intern Med.* 1992;116:798-805.

22-10. Ou CY, et al. Molecular epidemiology of HIV transmission in a dental practice. *Science.* 1992;256:1165-1171.

22-11. Hillis DM. Support for dental HIV transmission. *Nature.* 1994;369:24-25.

22-12. Altman LK. AIDS mystery that won't go away: did a dentist infect 6 patients? *New York Times.* July 5, 1994:B6.

22-13. Feldman RE. Hepatitis in dental professionals. *JAMA.* 1975;232:1222-1223.

22-14. Mosely JW, et al. Hepatitis B virus infection in dentists. *N Engl J Med.* 1975;293:729-734.

22-15. Smith JL, et al. Comparative risk of hepatitis B among physicians and dentists. *J Infect Dis.* 1976;133:715-716.

22-16. Mosley JW, et al. Viral hepatitis as an occupational hazard of dentists. *J Am Dent Assoc.* 1975;90:992-997.

22-17. Mori M. Status of viral hepatitis in the world community; its incidence amongst dentists and dental personnel. *Int Dent J.* 1984;34:11-5.

22-18. Smith HM, et al. Does screening high risk patients for hepatitis B virus protect dentists? *Br Med J.* 1986;295:309-310.

22-19. Gerbert B, et al. Possible health care professional-to-patient HIV transmission. *JAMA.* Apr 10, 1991;265(14);1845-1848.

22-20. Cendoroglo NM, et al. Environmental transmission of hepatitis B and hepatitis C viruses within the hemodialysis unit. *Artif Organs.* 1995 Mar;19(3):251-255.

22-21. HIV transmission in a dialysis center - Colombia, 1991-1993. *MMWR.* Jun 2, 1995;44(21):404-412.

22-22. Patient exposures to HIV during nuclear medicine procedures. *MMWR.* Aug 7 1992;41(31):575-578.

22-23. Recommended infection -control practices for dentistry, 1993. *MMWR.* May 28, 1993;42(No. RR-8):1-12.

22-24. Ahtone J, et al. Hepatitis B and dental personnel: transmission to patients and prevention issues. *J Am Dent Assoc.* 1983;106:219-222.

22-25. Hadler SC, et al. An outbreak of hepatitis B in a dental practice. *Ann Intern Med.* 1981;5:133-138.

22-26. Levin ML, et al. Hepatitis B transmission by dentists. *JAMA.* 1974;228:1139-1140.

22-27. Rimland D, et al. Hepatitis B outbreak traced to an oral surgeon. *N Engl J Med.* 1977;296:953-958.

22-28. Goodwin D, et al. An oral surgeon-related hepatitis B outbreak. *Calif Morbid.* 1976;14.

22-29. Reingold AL, et al. Transmission of hepatitis B by an oral surgeon. *J Infect Dis.* 1982;145:262-268.

22-30. Goodman RA, et al. Hepatitis B transmission from dental personnel to patients: unfinished business. *Ann Intern Med.* 1982;96:119.

22-31. Shaw FE, et al. Lethal outbreak of hepatitis B in a dental practice. *JAMA.* 1986;255:3261-3264.

22-32. Outbreak of hepatitis B associated with an oral surgeon, New Hampshire. *MMWR.* 1987;36:132-133.

22-33. Scully, C. Hepatitis B: An update in relation to dentistry. *British Dental J.* 1995;159:323.

22-34. Kent GP, et al. A large outbreak of acupuncture-associated hepatitis B. *Am J Epidemiol.* 1988;127:591-598.

22-35. Canter J, et al. An outbreak of hepatitis B associated with jet injections in a weight reduction clinic. *Arch Intern Med.* 1990;150:1923-1927.

22-36. Polish LB, et al. Nosocomial transmission of hepatitis B virus associated with the use of a spring-loaded finger-stick device. *N Engl J Med.* 1992;326:721-725.

22-37. Improper infection-control practices during employee vaccination programs - District of Columbia and Pennsylvania, 1993. *MMWR.* Dec 24, 1993;42(50):969-971.

22-38. Gerberding JL. The infected health care provider. *New Engl J Med.* 1996;334:594-595.

23. OPERAIDS

23-1. Jancin B. HIV, Other diseases pose rising threat to health professionals. *Internal Medicine News.* Feb 1, 1995:1,18.

23-2. Wright JG, et al. Mechanisms of glove tears and sharp injuries among surgical personnel. *JAMA.* 1991 Sep 25;266(12):1668-1671.

23-3. Palmer JD, et al. The mechanisms and risks of surgical glove perforation. *J Hosp Infect.* 1992 Dec;22(4):279-286.

23-4. Greco RJ, et al. Risk of blood contact through surgical gloves in aesthetic procedures. Aesthetic Plast Surg. 1993 Spring;17(2):167-168.

23-5. Hansen K, et al. Loss of glove integrity during common ED procedures. *Int Conf AIDS.* 1992 Jul 19-24;8(2):C336 (abstract no. PoC 4547).

23-6. Mast ST, et al. Efficacy of gloves in reducing blood volumes transferred during simulated needle-stick injury. *J Infect Dis.* 1993;168:1589-1592.

23-7. Mayhall CG. Risk factors for the Development of Surgical Site Infections. *Hospital Epidemiology and Infection Control.* Williams and Wilkins, Baltimore. 1996:157-160.

23-8. Bennett JV, et al. Intraoperative Events Influencing Infection Rates. *Hospital Infections.* 3rd Edition. Little, Brown and Company, Boston. 1992:692-694.

23-9. Hogue CW, et al. Potential toxicity from prolonged anesthesia: a case report of a thirty-hour anesthetic. *J Clin Anesth.* May/Jun 1990;2(3):183-187.

23-10. Hallmo P, et al. Laryngeal papillomatosis with human papillomavirus DNA contracted by a laser surgeon. *Eur Arch Otorhinolaryngol.* 1991;248(7):425-427.

23-11. Garden JM, et al. Papillomavirus in the vapor of carbon dioxide laser-treated verrucae. *JAMA.* 1988;259:1199-1202.

23-12. Wisniewski PM, et al. Studies on the transmission of viral disease via the CO2 laser plume and ejecta. *J Reprod Med.* 1990 Dec;35(12):1117-1123.

23-13. Robert LM, et al. HIV Transmission in the health-care setting: Risks to health-care workers and patients. *Infec Dis Clin of N Am.* Jun 1994;8(2): 319-330.

23-14. Health Care Worker Occupational Exposure to HIV. *International AIDS Society - USA.* June1994;2(1):1,10.

23-15. Kantrowitz B, et al. Doctors and AIDS. *Newsweek.* July 1, 1991:48-57.

23-16. Ippolito G, et al. The risk of occupational human immunodeficiency virus infection in health care workers. *Arch Intern Med.* June,1993;153:1451-1458.

23-17. High occupational exposure rate found among hospital personnel. *Internal Medicine World Report.* Feb 1995;10(3):1,18.

23-18. Powell J. Daddy has AIDS. *Good Housekeeping.* May 1995:96,216.

23-19. Aoun H. When a house officer gets AIDS. *N Engl J Med.* 1989;321:693-696.

23-20. Henderson DK, et al. Risk for occupational transmission of human immunodeficiency virus type 1 associated with clinical exposures. *Annals Intern Med.*1990;113(10):740-746.

23-21. Resnic F, et al. Occupational exposure among medical students and house staff at a New York City medical center. *Arch Intern Med.* Jan 9, 1995;155:75-80.

23-22. Recommendations for preventing transmission of human immunodeficiency virus and hepatitis B virus to patients during exposure-prone invasive procedures. *MMWR.* July 1991;40(No. RR-8):1-5.

23-23. Monmaney, T. Surgeon gave 19 patients hepatitis virus. *Los Angeles Times.* Feb 29, 1996:B10.

23-24. Harpaz R, et al. Transmission of hepatitis B virus to multiple patients from a surgeon without evidence of inadequate infection control. *N Engl J Med.* 1996;334:549-554.

23-25. Esteban JI, et al. Transmission of hepatitis C virus by a cardiac surgeon. *New Engl J Med.* 1996;334:555-560.

24. CALL IT WHAT YOU WANT!!

24-1. 1993 Revised classification system for HIV infection and expanded surveillance case definition for AIDS among adolescents and adults. *MMWR.* 1992;41:(no. RR-17).

24-2. Update: Impact of the expanded AIDS surveillance case definition for adolescents and adults on case reporting - United States, 1993. *MMWR.* Mar 11, 1994;43(9):160-170.

24-3. Update: Trends in AIDS diagnosis and reporting under the expanded surveillance definition for adolescents and adults - United States, 1993. *MMWR.* Nov 18, 1994;43(45):826-831.

24-4. Official Authorized Addenda: Human Immunodeficiency Virus Infection Codes and Official Guidelines for Coding and Reporting ICD-9-CM. *MMWR.* 1994;43(RR-12):13-15.

25. WE HAVE BASEBALL FOR THAT

25-1. The nation's prevention agency. *MMWR.* Nov 6, 1992;41(44):833.

25-2. Smith HM. The Deadly Politics of AIDS. *Wall Street Journal.* Oct 25, 1995.

25-3. HIV prevention through case management for HIV-infected persons - selected sites, United States, 1989-1992. *MMWR.* Jun 18, 1993;42(23):448-456.

25-4. Attitudes About HIV Reporting Among California's Public Health Officials. *California STD Control Association.* June 6, 1995:1-7.

25-5. Shilts R. *And The Band Played On.* St. Martin's Press, New York. 1987.

25-6. Assessment of laboratory reporting to supplement active AIDS surveillance-Colorado. *MMWR.* 1993;42:749-752.

25-7. Differences between anonymous and confidential registrants for HIV testing - Seattle, 1986-1992. *MMWR.* Jan 29, 1993;42(3):53-56.

25-8. Landis SE, et al. Results of a Randomized Trial of Partner Notification in Cases of HIV Infection in North Carolina. *N Engl J Med.* 326:101-106, 1992.

25-9. Rubinstien EM, et al. Testing of HIV-seropositive minority women. *The AIDS Reader.* Jan-Feb 1996;6(1):22-28.

25-10. Update: AIDS among women - United States, 1994. *MMWR.* 1995;44:81-84.

25-11. AIDS Among Racial/Ethnic Minorities - United States, 1993. *MMWR.* 1994;43(35):644-647.

25-12. Minkoff H, et al. Pediatric HIV disease, zidovudine in pregnancy and unblinding heelstick surveys. *JAMA.* Oct 1995;274(14):1165-1168.

25-13. Isaacman SC, et al. Neonatal HIV Seroprevalence Studies: A critique of national and international practices. *J Legal Medicine.* 14:413-461.

25-14. Roy B. The Tuskegee syphilis experiment: biotechnology and the administrative state. *J Natl Med Assoc.* 1995 Jan;87(1):56-67.

25-15. Thomas SB, et al. The Tuskegee syphilis study, 1932 to 1972: implications for HIV education and AIDS risk education programs in the black community. *Am J Public Health.* Nov 1991;81(11):1498-1505.

25-16. Caplan AL. Twenty years after. The legacy of the Tuskegee syphilis study. When evil intrudes. *Hastings Cent Rep.* Nov-Dec 1992;22(6):29-32.

25-17. Harris JC. Why Not Include Contact Tracing in HIV Prevention? *Annals Int Med.* 1994;121(5):388.

25-18. Kettinger L, et al. Public Health uses of HIV-infection reports - So Carolina, 1986-1991. *MMWR.* Apr 17, 1992;41(15):245-249.

25-19. Hinman AR. Strategies to prevent HIV infection in the United States. *Am J Pub Health.* Dec 1991;81(12):1557-1559.

25-20. Department of Defense Appropriations for 1970. *Hearings before a Subcommittee of the Committee on Appropriations House of Representatives Ninety-First Congress, First session.* George H. Mahon, Texas, Chairman. H.B. 15090. Synthetic Biological Agents.

25-21. Weiss R. Of myths and mischief. *Discover.* Dec 1994;15(12):36-42.

26. PLANES, TRAINS, AND TUBERCULAIDS

26-1. Gostin LG. Controlling the resurgent tuberculosis epidemic. *JAMA.* Jan 13, 1993;269(2):255-261.

26-2. Raviglione MC, et al. Global epidemiology of tuberculosis: morbidity and mortality of a worldwide epidemic. *JAMA.* 1995;273:220-226.

26-3. Death from tuberculosis reach historic levels; 3 million died in 1995. *Infectious Disease News.* May 1996;9(5):9.

26-4. Finkelstein JB. Global Emergency: Tuberculosis is killing more people than ever. *Internal Medicine News.* May 15, 1996;29(10):43.

26-5.   Burwen DR, et al. National trends in the concurrence of Tuberculosis and acquired immunodeficiency syndrome. *Arch Intern Med.* 1995;155:1281-1286.

26-6.   Ball S, et al. Tuberculosis and its management in patients with HIV disease. *The AIDS Reader.* Dec 1994;4(6):181-192.

26-7.   Haas DW, et al. Tuberculosis in patients with HIV infection. *Opportunistic Infections of AIDS.* Publication of Vanderbilt University, School of Medicine, 1994:14-23.

26-8.   Tuberculosis Management. *International AIDS Society-USA.* Aug 1994;2(2):13-15.

26-9.   Laraque F, et al. Tuberculosis in HIV-Infected Patients. *The AIDS Reader.* Sept/Oct 1992;2:171-180.

26-10.   Eriki PP, et al. The influence of human immunodeficiency virus infection on tuberculosis in Kampala, Uganda. *Am Rev Respir Dis.* 1991;143:185-187.

26-11.   DeCock KM, et al. Risk of tuberculosis in patients with HIV-1 and HIV-11 infections on Abidjan, Ivory Coast. *Brit Med J.* 1991;302:496-504.

26-12.   Gordin FM. Impact of HIV infection on the epidemiology, natural history, and diagnosis of tuberculosis. *Opportunistic Complications of HIV.* 1994;3(2):32-35.

26-13.   Comstock GW, et al. Can we control TB this time? *Patient Care.* May 15, 1995:97-117.

26-14.   Sepkowitz KA. AIDS, Tuberculosis, and the health care worker. *Clin Infect Dis.* 1995;20:232-242.

26-15.   Charnow JA. Pediatrician may have exposed children to TB. Potential exposure at a hospital in a Pennsylvania city leads to skin testing of 1,432 children. *Infectious Disease News.* May 1996;9(5):8-9.

26-16.   Barnes PF, et al. Transmission of tuberculosis among the urban homeless. *JAMA.* Jan. 24/31, 1996;275(4):305-308.

26-17.   Friedman LN, et al. Tuberculosis, AIDS, and death among substance abusers on welfare in New York City. *New Engl J Med.* Mar 28, 1996;334(13):828-833.

26-18.   Alland D, et al. Transmission of tuberculosis in New York City. *N Engl J Med.* 1992;330:1710-1716.

26-19.   Edlin BR, et al. An outbreak of multidrug-resistant tuberculosis among hospitalized patients with the acquired immunodeficiency syndroms. *N Engl J Med.* 1992;326:1514-1521.

26-20.   Reichman LB. Multidrug-resistant tuberculosis: meeting the challenge. *Hospital Practice.* May 15, 1994;29(5):85-96.

26-21.   Fischl MA, et al. An Outbreak of tuberculosis caused by multiple-drug-resistant tubercle bacilli among patients with HIV infection. *Annals of Internal Medicine.* 1992;117:177-183.

26-22.   Kocs D, et al. Tuberculosis treatment in developing nations. *JAMA.* (letters) July 12, 1995;274(2):125.

26-23.   Driver CR, et al. Transmission of Mycobacterium tuberculosis associated with air travel. *JAMA.* 1994;272:1031-1035.

26-24.   Wenzel RP. Airline travel and infection. *New Engl J Med.* Apr 11, 1996;334(15):981-982.

26-25.   Kenyon TA, et al. Transmission of multidrug-resistant Mycobacterium Tuberculosis during a long airplane flight. *New Engl J Med.* Apr 11,

1996;334(15):934-938.

26-26. Adams DS, et al. Transmission and control of caprine arthritis-encephalitis virus. *Am J Vet Res.* 1983;44:1670-1676.

26-27. Phelps S, et al. Caprine arthritis-encephalitis virus infection. *J Vet Med Assoc.* Dec 15, 1993;203(12):1663-1666.

26-28. McGuire TC, et al. Caprine arthritis encephalitis lentivirus transmission and disease. *Curr Top Microbiol Immunol.* 1990;160:61-75.

26-29. Yamamoto JK. et al. Epidemiologic and clinical aspects of feline immunodeficiency virus infection in cats from the continental United States and Canada and possible mode of transmission. *J Am Vet Med Assoc.* 1989;194:213.

27. A FOOL AND HIS MONEY

27-1. Oldham, J. The Economic Cost of AIDS. *Los Angeles Times.* Oct 13, 1995:D1.

27-2. Lifetime HIV care for children averages $418.63. *Infectious Disease News.* Apr 1996;9(4):12.

27-3. Hanvelt RA, et al. Indirect costs of HIV/AIDS mortality in Canada. *AIDS.* 1994;8:F7-F11.

27-4. Dobkin JF. AIDS and the public hospital crisis. *Infect Med.* 1995;12(9):412.

27-5. Saillant C. Another AIDS setback? *Ventura Star Free Press.* Mar 2, 1996;A1, A6.

27-6. Owens DK, et al. Screening surgeons for HIV infection, a cost-effectiveness analysis. *Ann of Int Med.* 1995 May;122(9):641-652.

27-7. Chavey WE, et al. Cost-effectivenes analysis of screening health care workers for HIV. *J Fam Pract.* 1994;38:249-257.

27-8. Mandel ID, The diagnostic uses of saliva. *J Oral Pathol Med.* 1990 Mar;19(3):119-125.

27-9. Chamnanput J, et al. Comparison of eight commercial test kits for detecting anti-HIV antibodies in saliva specimens. *AIDS.* 1993;7:1026.

27-10. Hurtado LV, et al. Searching for anti-HIV antibodies in saliva samples. *Int Conf AIDS.* 1994 Aug 7-12;10(1):229 (abstract no. PB0346).

27-11. Francois-Gerard C, et al. Multicenter European evaluation of HIV testing on serum and saliva samples. *Int Conf AIDS.* 1993 Jun 6-11;9(2):766 (abstract no. PO-C31-3293).

27-12. Spielberg F, et al. HIV EIA testing of saliva and urine under tropical conditions. *Natl Conf Hum Retroviruses Relat Infect (2nd).* 1995 Jan 29-Feb 2:120.

27-13. Frerichs RR, et al. Comparison of saliva and serum for HIV surveillance in developing countries. *Lancet.* 1992;340:1496-1499.

27-14. Frerichs RR. Personal screening for HIV in developing countries. *Lancet.* Apr 16, 1994;343:960-962.

27-15. Brown LR, et al. *Vital Signs 1996.* Worldwatch Institute. W.W. Norton and Company, New York. 1996.

28. 6,000 TIMES WORSE

28-1. Outbreak of Ebola viral hemorrhagic fever - Zaire, 1995. *MMWR.* May 19, 1995;44(19):381-382.

28-2. Mandell GL, et al. *Principles and Practice of Infectious Diseases.* John Wiley and Sons, New York. 1985.

28-3.   Cowley G, et al. Outbreak of Fear. *Newsweek*. May 22, 1995:48-55.

28-4.   Preston R. *The Hot Zone*. Random House, New York. 1994.

28-5.   Heymann DL, et al. Ebola hemorrhagic fever; Tandala, Zaire, 1977-1978. *J Infect Dis*. 1980;142:372.

28-6.   Dowell SF. Ebola hemorrhagic fever: why were children spared? *Pediatr Infect Dis J*. 1996;15:189-191.

28-7.   Nkowane B. Prevalence and incidence of HIV infection in Africa: A review of data published in 1990. *AIDS*. 1991;5 (suppl 1):S7-15.

29.   N B AIDS

29-1.   Wulf S. As if by Magic. *Time*. Feb 12, 1996;147(7):58-62.

29-2.   Belongia EA, et al. An outbreak of herpes gladiatorum at a high-school wrestling camp. *New Engl J Med*. Sept 26, 1991;325(13):906-910.

29-3.   Mast EE, et al.. Transmission of blood-borne pathogens during sports: risk and prevention. *Ann Intern Med*. 1995;122:283-285.

29-4.   Karjalainen J. Blood-borne Pathogens in Sports. Letter to the Editor., *Ann Intern Med*. Oct 15, 1995;123(8): 635-636.

29-5.   Berg R, et al. Australia antigen in hepatitis among Swedish track-finders. *Acta Pathol Microbiol Scand*. 1971;79:423-427.

29-6.   Ringertz O, et al. Serum hepatitis among Swedish track-finders. An epidemiologic study. *N Engl J Med*. 1967;276:540-546.

29-7.   Torre D, et al. Transmission of HIV-I infection via sports injury. *Lancet*. May 1990;335:1105.

29-8.   O'Farrel N, et al. Transmission of HIV-I infection after a fight. *Lancet*. 1992;339:246.

29-9.   Ippolito G, et al. Transmission of zidovudine-resistant HIV during a bloody fight. *JAMA*. Aug 1994;272(6):433-434.

29-10.   Loveday C. HIV disease and sport. *Lancet*. Jun 23, 1990;335:1532.

29-11.   Louganis, G. *Breaking the Surface*. Random House, New York. 1995.

29-12.   Springer S. Boxer's HIV test heats up debate over risk to others. *Los Angeles Times*. Feb 13, 1996:A1,A9.

29-13.   Springer S. HIV testing to be proposed. *Los Angeles Times*. Feb 14, 1996:C1, C10.

32.   HEALER OR ACCOMPLICE?

32-1.   Dal Porto RM. Say good-bye to your civil rights. *Being Alive. People with HIV/AIDS Action Coalition Newsletter*. April 1994:8.

32-2.   SCPIE Risk Management Publication. Reporting Child Abuse. *Safe Practice*. Aug 1995;1(2):1-2.

33.   LITIGAIDS: *The Right To Be Dead Right!*

33-1.   Verner, LJ. "Philadelphia" Story. *HIV Hotline*. June-July 1994;4:2.

33-2.   1994 Fall headcount for JD programs at University of California schools. Office of the Assistant Vice President for Planning, University of CA, Office of the President. Oakland, CA. Personal Communication.

33-3.   Shuit DP. Cuts pose threat to AIDS programs, county workers say. *Los Angeles Times*. Aug 19, 1995:B3.

33-4.   *California Health and Safety Code*. Section 199.21and 199.37 (unauthorized disclosure of HIV).

33-5.   Wecht DN, et al. Legal aspects of AIDS and the practice of medicine: An update. *Legal Medicine Perspectives.* Winter 1992;1(1):1, 4-7.

33-6.   Gostin LO. Liability Risks. *PAACNOTES.* Oct 1992;4:312-314.

33-7.   Vener, LJ. The Attorney's corner. *HIV Hotline.* Feb/Mar 1994;4(2):3.

33-8.   Between a Rock and a Hard Place: AIDS and the Conflicting Physician's Duties of Preventing Disease Transmission and Safeguarding Confidentiality (1987) *76 Georgetown Law Journal 169.*

33-9.   AIDS: Balancing the Physician's Duty to Warn and Confidentiality Concerns (1989) *38 Emory Law Journal 279.*

33-10. Hugh Grant. *Los Angeles Times.* (series of articles) June 1995.

33-11. Testing donors or organs, tissues, and semen for antibody to human T-lymphotropic virus type III/lymphadenopathy-associated virus. *MMWR.* 1985;34:294.

33-12. Chiasson MA, et al. Human immunodeficiency virus transmission through artificial insemination. *J Acquir Immune Defic Syndr.* 1990;3:69-72.

33-13. Joseph SC. *Dragon Within the Gates.* Carroll and Graf, New York. 1992.

33-14. CDC guidelines for preventing transmission of human immunodeficiency virus through transplantation of human tissue and organs. *MMWR.* 1994;43(No RR-8):1-17.

33-15. Howard, PK. *The Death of Common Sense.* Random House, New York. 1995.

35. ACROSS THE STREET FROM DISNEYLAND

35-1.   Shuit DP. State Doctors Group Urges HIV Reporting. *Los Angeles Times.* Mar 7, 1995:A1,A16.

35-2.   Ocampo RA, *NEWS for Immediate Release* from the California Medical Association News Bureau, March 7, 1995.

35-3.   Shuit, DP. Doctors in state rescind policy on reporting HIV. *Los Angeles Times.* Mar 6, 1996:A1, A12.

35-4.   Nary GO, et al. Defusing a Global Time Bomb! *PAACNOTES.* 1992;4:190-191.

35-5.   Miller J. AIDS Ten Years After: the signs of strain, discouragement and battle fatigue are everywhere. *UCSF Magazine.* Feb 1994;15(1):1-22.

35-6.   Centers for Disease Control. World AIDS Day - December 1, 1993. *MMWR.* Nov 19, 1993;42(45):869.

35-7.   Kubetin SK. Prevalence of HIV is uncertain. *Internal Medicine News.* Mar 15, 1996;29(6):27.

35-8.   Barnett T. *AIDS in Africa: Its Present and Future Impact.* London, Bellhaven Press. 1992.

35-9.   Mann J. *AIDS in the World.* Cambridge, Mass: Harvard University Press. 1992.

36. POINT OF NO RETURN

36-1.   HIV seroprevalence among adults treated for cardiac arrest before reaching a medical facility - Seattle, Washington, 1989-1990. *MMWR.* May 29, 1992;47(21):381-383.

36-2.   Murray P. *Manual of Clinical Microbiology.* 6th ed. Washington, D.C., ASM Press. 1995.

37. WHERE THE RUBBER MEETS THE ROAD
What I Tell My Children

37-1.   The Daedalus Project AIDS Benefit 1995. Oregon Shakespeare Festival, August 14, 1995.

INDEX

Bay Area Newly Described Acquired
Immune Disorder. *See* BANDAID
Bergalis, Kimberly, 106
Biaxin, 58
Blinded AIDS surveillance, 125
Blood-splash injury, 108, 113, 147,
149, 185
Bombay brothels, 176
Boxing, HIV testing of professional
boxers, 149
Branched DNA testing, 56
Bush, President George, 147

—C—

California Assembly Bill (AB403), 163
California Department of Health
Services Office of AIDS, 97
California law (section 11166 of the
penal code), 159
California Medical Association (CMA),
175
Candidiasis, 58, 120
Castro District, San Francisco, 29
CCR-5 gene, 64
CD4, 36, 42, 45, 65, 67, 78, 100, 120,
121, 162
CDC, 74, 82
recommendations for prevention of HIV
in dentistry, 103
CDC guidelines redefining AIDS, 126
Cellular immunity, 67. *See* cytotoxic
T-lymphocyte immune response
Centers for Disease Control and
Prevention. *See* CDC
Chancroid, 95
Chimpanzees, 65
Chlamydia, 95
Chopin, 129
Civil libertarians, 13, 40, 75, 108,
117, 160
CMV, 57, 96. *See also*
cytomegalovirus
Coccidioidiomycosis, 120
Colorado
HIV reporting laws challenged, 124
Columbia
HIV transmission during hemodialysis,
103
Communitarian thought, 93
Condoms and HIV transmission, 91
Continuing medical education (CME),
164
Cost of treating all Americans with
HIV, 140
Cryptococcus, 20, 45, 58, 69, 78, 120

Cryptosporidia, 58
Cuba, 38, 39, 40
Cytomegalovirus, 57, 96, 120, 136
Cytotoxic T-lymphocyte immune
response in Gambian prostitutes,
64

—D—

D4T. *See* nucleoside antiretrovirals
Daedalus Project, Ashland Oregon,
182
DDC. *See* reverse transcriptase
inhibitors
DDI. *See* reverse transcriptase
inhibitors
Declaration of Geneva 1948, 126
Declaration of Helsinki, 126
Declaration of Prevention, 177
Dental Associations
recommendations to HIV-positive
dental workers, 104
Dental procedures
and hepatitis B outbreaks, 102
Diflucan, 58
Dinosaur, 17
Disneyland, 175
Disseminated intravascular
coagulation (DIC), 142
Dream Team, 68
Dugas, Gaeten
patient "Zero", 69

—E—

Early investigational drug trials, 53
Ebola, 50, 59, 141, 142, 143, 144
EBV. *See* Epstein-Barr Virus
Epidemiology, 82, 106, 111, 153, 175
Epidemiology,
definition, 27
Epivir, 57, 146. *See also* 3TC
Epogen, 59
Epstein-Barr Virus, 96
Etzioni, Amitai, 93

—F—

FDA. *See* Food and Drug
Administration
Federal Centers for Disease Control
AIDS classification. *See also* CDC
Feminists, 125
Florida Department of Health and
Rehabilitative Services, 106
Food and Drug Administration, 50,
54, 56, 57, 154
Foreman, George, 51

Universal precautions, 111, 113, 116
Universal screening, 72, 75, 76, 124, 173
University of California law school enrollment, 163
University of California, San Francisco General Hospital, 30
Urine test for HIV, 138
Utah Jazz, 145

—V—

Vancouver, Canada
    International AIDS Conference, 177
Varese, Italy
    HIV transmission between soccer players, 146
Venereal warts. *See* papilloma virus
Viral amplification, 66
Viral load, 56, 59, 66, 67
    cost of test, 136

—W—

Wallace, Mike, 106
Walters, Barbara, 150
Wasting syndrome. *See* severe wasting

West Hollywood, 102
WHO. *See* World Health Organization
Window period, 117, 173, 184
World Health Organization, 74, 76
    annual STD estimates, 95
    children with HIV, projection for year 2000, 37
    HIV prediction by year 2000, 176
Wyoming, Thermopolis, 107

—X—

Xenografting, 66. *See* also baboon bone marrow

—Y—

Yeltsin, Boris, 86
Yokohama, Japan
    International AIDS Conference, 177

—Z—

Zaire, 69
    Ebola deaths, 141
    HIV deaths, 141
Zidovudine. *See* AZT
Zithromax, 58
Zovirax. *See* acyclovir

All truth passes through three steps.
First, it is ridiculed.
Second, it is violently opposed.
Third, it is accepted as being self-evident.

— *Arthur Schopenhauer*

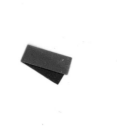